The Rice Diet
Renewal

The Rice Diet Renewal

A Healing 30-Day Program for Lasting Weight Loss

Kitty Gurkin Rosati,
M.S., R.D., L.D.N.

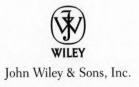

WILEY

John Wiley & Sons, Inc.

Published by John Wiley & Sons, Inc., Hoboken, New Jersey
Published simultaneously in Canada

Pages 120–121: The Positivity Self Test reprinted with the permission of Barbara Fredrickson; pages 18–19: "Sailing from Cape Fear to Hope Island" reprinted with the permission of "Charles."

The information contained in this book is not intended to serve as a replacement for professional medical advice. Any use of the information in this book is at the reader's discretion. The author and the publisher specifically disclaim any and all liability arising directly or indirectly from the use or application of any information contained in this book. A health care professional should be consulted regarding your specific situation.

For general information about our other products and services, please contact our Customer Care Department within the United States at (800) 762-2974, outside the United States at (317) 572-3993 or fax (317) 572-4002.

Wiley also publishes its books in a variety of electronic formats. Some content that appears in print may not be available in electronic books. For more information about Wiley products, visit our web site at www.wiley.com.

Library of Congress Cataloging-in-Publication Data:

Rosati, Kitty Gurkin, date.
  The rice diet renewal : a healing 30-day program for lasting weight loss / Kitty Gurkin Rosati.
        p. cm.
    Includes bibliographical references and index,
      ISBN 978-0-470-52544-9 (cloth); ISBN 978-0-470-61585-0 (ebk.);
ISBN 978-0-470-61586-7 (ebk.); ISBN 978-0-470-61588-1 (ebk.)
    1. Reducing diets. 2. Cookery (Rice) 3. High-carbohydrate diet.
I. Title.
      RM222.2.R6463   2010
      613.2'5—dc22   2010006817

Printed in the United States of America

10 9 8 7 6 5 4 3 2 1

A Note to the Reader

It is important to check with your physician prior to beginning any diet, especially if you are taking any medications. Due to the rapid weight loss with the Rice Diet, it is important to consult with your physician before reducing your fat, sodium, and calories. You may be on medication that will need to be altered or discontinued before changing your diet, and your doctor is the best person to help you do this. Do not make any changes in your medication regimen without your physician's advice. Since many physicians and health care professionals are unfamiliar with the impact of a truly low-sodium diet, you should point out the low sodium content of the Rice Diet to your doctor. Feel free, as well, to refer your physician to the Rice Diet Clinic, and we will be happy to be of assistance. We can be reached at www.ricediet.com. We also recommend that you keep a record of your weight, any heart disease risk factors, and any other health predictors that you are aware of having.

Contents

Acknowledgments

On this seventy-year anniversary of the Rice Diet Program, my heart is filled with gratitude for all who have contributed and participated in this unique approach to healing. From our founder, Dr. Walter Kempner, who passed the torch to our director, our cardiologist, and my husband, Dr. Robert Rosati; to our poet in residence and endocrinologist, Dr. Frank Neelon; and to our amazing dietitians, interns, consulting practitioners, secretaries, and kitchen staff, I give thanks. My deep appreciation goes to Jayne Charles, Judy Rivers, and Betsy Hamilton, who answer the phone calls and e-mails of the public; to our dietitians, especially Anna LaBarre, Ryan Sobus, Cece Eckert, Maura Lairson, and Sarah Jones; to the kitchen staff's loving touch in creating delicious meals from locally grown, organic ingredients—these culinary artists include Nancy Navarro, Derek Treuer, Cassandra Davis, Raheem Huggins, and many other loving people. Thanks to all of our staff members, who feed us on so many different levels, nurturing the physical, emotional, mental, and spiritual health not only of the Ricer community here, but also of the growing numbers of readers who have learned this *dieta* at home. May blessings abound for them and for everyone who is committed to inspiring others to make the most of their gifts, to seek true health, and to live their lives to the fullest.

This book can stretch us to heal ourselves by grappling with the root of our issues. It can catapult and sustain the changes we make to our health and our lives. The book is greatly enriched by the addition of true healing stories provided by our Ricer community and from my own life and family. All of these stories are true; they are not composites that we created to exaggerate or embellish a story. I have found truth to be more transformative than fiction, so only the names have been changed. I commend those who have shared their stories for "showing up" for themselves and choosing to "make a difference" with their lives. I am forever grateful to everyone who bravely shared his or her truth with the hope and intention of helping others, who in turn will pay it forward and inspire yet more people to embrace the health rewards of the Rice *dieta*.

Many sojourners who are gifted in healing and various practitioners of energy medicine have graced our grounds and my life; my appreciation for them is beyond measure. It is one of my greatest joys and marvels to experience and share in what has been called inner healing, or the healing of memories that affect not only our past but also our future health. Special thanks to these gifted souls, from Reverend Tommy Tyson to Karen Winstead, Todd Brazee, Larry Burk, and Carolyn Craft. Although my spiritual mentor described his healing abilities as a gift of healing from God, I have personally witnessed and benefited from other practitioners who call their energetic approaches to healing axiatonal therapy, breath therapy, emotional freedom technique, and Hakomi therapy. The multisensorial approaches to healing that have come into my life during this book's gestation have greatly blessed me; I'm sure that Little Windows' music and Wendy Whitson's paintings will touch you deeply as well. Sharing in these two creative processes was indeed among the highlights of the last few years for me.

Every book, like every newborn, has a unique conception, gestation, and delivery—unlike any other that has come before. This book, my fourth, illustrates this metaphor almost comically. The breadth of this book's being was so vast that it became clear that all preconceived notions were just that! But thanks to my agent, Loretta Barrett, and my editors, Christel Winkler, Tom Miller, and Kimberly Monroe-Hill, the book was birthed as it was meant to be and right on time. Praise be to God!

Last and foremost, I will forever be grateful to my husband and my son, who allow me the flexibility of keeping an unpredictable and sometimes bizarre schedule as a writer and who accept my creative inspirations and visions. And right behind my immediate family is my deepest appreciation for my collaborator, Billie Fitzpatrick, who after our three books together knows my head and my heart as well as anyone does. Thank you, God, for gifting Billie with the patience and tenacity to assist me with the birthing of this one!

Introduction

For the last nineteen years, I have had the great pleasure and privilege of teaching and learning about healing at the Rice Diet Program in Durham, North Carolina. Participants here, fondly nicknamed Ricers, have the opportunity to experience the fastest, safest, and most effective way to lose weight and improve every other modifiable risk factor of heart disease and, in fact, most diseases. Founded in 1939, the Rice Diet Program has for seventy years facilitated and collected the most impressive weight-loss and weight-maintenance data and heart disease risk-factor improvements that have ever been documented. Men each lose an average of thirty pounds and women an average of nineteen pounds in the first month on the program. But what is even more impressive is the long-term success of our thousands of participants: 43 percent of Ricers have maintained their weight loss or lost even more after six years back home! Our founder, Dr. Walter Kempner, often said, as Nietzsche had previously and similarly stated many years earlier, "It's not the intensity of the great passion, but the duration of the great passion that makes a great man [and woman] great!"

These encouraging—some people think near-miraculous—statistics are definitely a consequence of our world-famous Rice Diet, a low-sodium, low-fat eating plan made up of whole grains, beans, fruits, vegetables, and minimal animal protein. Yet the incredible number of pounds lost by Ricers from around the globe, the years that their weight loss has been maintained, and the fact that these people have restored their health after suffering from a wide variety of diseases are also the result of the integrated mind-body tools and practices that the Rice Diet Program encompasses. These practical exercises and experiential tools make up the four steps of *The Rice Diet Solution* and *The Rice Diet Cookbook*. The first step is the diet itself, which enables you to lose weight safely and quickly; the second step, becoming a mindful eater, takes you inside yourself so that you can become more conscious of how, why, and what you are eating; step three, taking time for yourself—whether it be time to exercise, do yoga, or meditate—gives you permission and space to be more in tune with a deeper part of yourself; and finally, step four, creating a community, asks that you reach out to other like-minded people to support and encourage your new way of life.

These simple steps inspired an enormous response from our readers and participants, far and wide. In hundreds of e-mails and one-on-one encounters, Ricers told us that these steps were at the crux of their ability to stick to the diet at home. The mind-body techniques gave them encouragement and inner confidence to maintain the changes to their lifestyles and helped them fully engage their bodies and their minds so that they could live in a fuller, more satisfying way. Ricers, whether they had come to the program here in Durham or had practiced the plan at home, seemed to grasp the radical difference between a restrictive *diet*, versus a *dieta*, the original Greek word that means "way of life." We hear story after story describing people's transformations. As Martine wrote to us on the Rice Diet forum (www.ricediet.com), she had always thought that the Rice Diet was simply a way to lose a lot of weight, fast. Then,

> A friend told me about the Rice Diet and I got your book. I was really impressed with the small emphasis on the "diet" and the large emphasis on the "changing your life."
>
> I began the Rice *Dieta*. After only a few days, once the salt, sugar, and refined carbs were out of my system, the cravings went away. Being a definite food addict, I know that abstinence from those things is the only way to eliminate craving. Then, as I matured spiritually, I realized that it was no longer okay to have twenty years of sobriety and keep eating while I was celebrating all that recovery. I have become so "aware" since starting this way of life. I feel feelings. I act honestly. I share with others. I thank God for this way of life. I am responsible. It is a choice. And I have never felt better. I am giving myself a chance to live. To grow. To be a part of life. And I owe all of it to the Rice *Dieta*. It has taught me much, much more than how to lose weight.

Martine is not alone. She is one of hundreds who have contacted us wanting more—*more* ways to connect to the underlying food and eating issues that have plagued them; *more* suggestions for how to dig deep and replace negative, powerless thinking with a confidence-boosting, self-loving credo; *more* exercises and tools that show them how to keep living the diet in a mindful, emotional, spiritual way.

As a result, the program has grown in this direction. Our roots are delving deeper, and our branches are reaching new heights and dimensions. In response, more and more experientials have evolved, mini-workshops that make the mind-body connection real, tangible, and practical. Utilizing the most current research from various sectors of science and art, including quantum physics, energetic healing methods, music and aromatherapy experientials, movies, and more, we expanded and deepened the mind-body steps of the original *Rice Diet Solution*. Thus, *The Rice Diet Renewal* was born.

We've discovered that when people practice these exercises and tools, they not only lose more weight and maintain their weight loss, but they also feel truly transformed—mind, body, and soul. They reach states of enlightenment and peace; they come to a more measured and accepting understanding of themselves and others; they find more loving rewards in their relationships; they are able to achieve more in their work and professional pursuits. In other words, when they become more physically free of overweight, clear of mind, and liberated from encumbering emotional baggage, they not only embody health, their most sought-after dreams and desires suddenly seem within reach. They become powerful. Or, more accurately, they step into the power that is already within.

My vision for this book is to reach and inspire the millions who are ready to actualize their greatest passions and thus succeed in finally achieving and maintaining their desired goals. Manifesting those dreams begins with understanding and then embracing your true health. Although *The Rice Diet Renewal* will show you how to lose weight safely for the long term and how to reverse chronic disease (including diabetes, heart disease, and its precursors), most important, it will inspire you to align your physical, mental, emotional, and spiritual selves so that you can actualize your true purpose and simply enjoy being you.

The Rice Diet Renewal promises to give you a path to true health. What do I mean by true health? Physical health that enables movement, agility, and an abundance of energy. Mental health that is marked by increased clarity of mind, purity of focus, and a renewed ability to set goals . . . and attain them. Emotional health that stems from being in touch with your feelings, enabling you to attend to your pains and fears, thus breaking the powerful and often negative cycle between unexpressed feelings and disease or illness, which is key to being free to be the person you aspire to be. And ultimately, spiritual health that enables you to celebrate love and co-create your life at the highest level. The Rice Diet Renewal is a practical program that you can follow and live every day; it is also a journey, one that will lead you on a path of inner healing, to a bountiful life full of purpose.

The connection between your mental, emotional, and spiritual well-being and your physical health is not only powerful, it's an essential priority if you truly want to achieve a life of happiness, enriched by your ability to reach your goals, love the people in your life, and celebrate the very essence of yourself.

How This Book Works

The Rice Diet Renewal offers thirty days of practical experientials, or exercises, that will revitalize and strengthen your body and soul—and all that lies in between. It will inspire a synergistic shift in your way of being and a new understanding of your true self because it brings together every aspect of who you are: your body, your mind, your heart, and your spirit or soul. True health—or healing—comes about and is sustained only if these four quadrants of your being are nurtured, integrated, and activated.

As you begin this journey, you will answer some questions about the way you think about your own health. You may learn that you take your health for granted. You may learn that you are often not attuned to your body's symptoms or cries for help or its immense and wonderful power to give you energy, enthusiasm, and creative juice. In part one, "Creating True Health," you will learn how to trace the connection between your body, your mind, your heart, and ultimately your soul, or spirit. Chapter 1, "Are You Ready for True Health?" invites you to consider the true meaning of health and how it is not restricted to the body—but it often begins there. If you want to heal, lose weight, or prevent or reverse disease, you need to start with cleansing your body, but you also need to address your mind (your thoughts and attitudes and patterns of behavior), your heart (your emotional issues, beginning with your relationship with food), and finally your spirit (by engaging your creative source or truth). In chapter 2, "Cleansing Your Body," you will learn how to detox your body, beginning with reducing the amount of sodium, fat, and processed foods in your diet. Following a simplified and modified version of the original

Rice Diet, you will eat whole grains, fruits, vegetables, legumes, dairy, and seafood, with occasional lean meat if desired.

Chapter 3, "Healing Your Heart," guides and inspires you to become aware of your feelings and any emotional scars you may have, so that you stop eating for emotional reasons and instead maximize the emotional experiences that empower you. You will learn specific techniques that have proved effective for many people, such as de-circuiting emotional eating by enhancing your awareness of why, what, when, where, and how you have historically coped by using food, rather than by dealing with the root of an emotional issue. You will also be invited to play the "Responsibility Game" and join the many others who have accepted the challenge to take on their lives as if they really matter!

In chapter 4, "Empowering Your Mind," you will learn about the latest well-documented research on quantum physics and the human brain, which boils down to the empowering reality that your thoughts matter. What you think and feel about your thoughts has a more powerful influence on your life than most people have ever imagined. When you can tap into the power of your brain in this way, you can reshape how you think about food and what you want to eat, and you actually awaken to the why, when, and where you do so. In other words, you gain access to control, or conscious choice, in a completely natural, effortless way. Once you experience this mental shift in awareness, you enhance your desire, focus, and power to exercise consciousness in all areas of your life, thus becoming more and more effective at actualizing your dreams.

Chapter 5, "Connecting with Your Spirit," invites you to reengage with your spiritual core, whether through yoga, prayer, meditation, or community outreach activities. The more you feel an interconnectedness with your Creator, the Universe—human, animal, plant, air, sea, and earth—the more your soul's center is able to realign and speak to you from its deep reservoir of peace and knowingness. What so many Ricers and I have found is that the more spiritually connected you feel—the more you love yourself, others, and your community—the more you can co-create your health and actualize your purpose.

The four integrated levels of healing, all of which are supported by research and are multisensory by nature, work to synergize your weight loss and overall physical wellness by enhancing mental clarity, emotional healing, and spiritual renewal. Inevitably and organically, this synergy leads to an awakening of your spirit, which is often described as a real experience of oneness with your fellow men and women and the creative force in the world at large. In this way, you will heal at the very core of your being, so that you not only free yourself from overweight, pain, and ill health, but you also discover, commit to, and manifest your biggest dreams and most important goals.

Again, in order to truly heal at your deepest level, you need to engage your body, heart, mind, and spirit—the four levels of your being—in a constant, day-by-day fashion. I've gathered and created practical exercises and tools and presented them in a thirty-day calendar, which you will be able to use in order to manifest your desire for true health. Although each exercise corresponds to a specific point in each chapter, the exercises themselves often apply to more than one level of healing. Thus, the tools can be used in many different ways, and you can do as many or as few as you wish, in whichever order makes the most sense to you.

Part two, "A Deeper Sense of True Health," opens the windows onto an even broader, deeper sense of true health. Chapter 6, "Conscious Consumption," introduces you to a conscious way of eating so that your food choices are healthy not only for your body but also for your heart, mind, and soul, as well as for the Universe. Have you ever heard of the slow food movement? Have you looked beyond organic to the beauty in biodynamic farming? You will see how some of the most profound thinkers of this generation are finding spiritual revitalization through their food choices and are transforming their lives via conscious consumption. You will become equipped and will desire to view your food choices through a wide-angle lens, knowing how your food is treated before it reaches your table, how genetically engineered and other nonorganic foods harm your health and damage the environment, and how you can become a significant part of the solution.

And finally, in chapter 7, "Amazing, Miraculous, and Extraordinary Healing," you will walk outside the fringes of the mainstream and experience firsthand how some people, including myself, have healed from all sorts of illnesses and conditions—of the body, the mind, and the heart—through spiritual pursuits and energy medicine. I, too, have experienced extraordinary healing; I returned from a near-death experience and healed from disorders that were described as incurable. Since that time, I have been totally committed to inspiring others to take full responsibility for their health and lives, with a *dieta*, or way of life, that prioritizes inner healing. I personally know and have witnessed in many others the profound ability that we all have been given to co-create our lives beyond our wildest imaginings.

This book is about much more than improving your health; it will inspire you to actualize your life. There are few things as satisfying and motivating as being and co-creating who and what you want to be and do. To feel that you are on time and right where you need to be, to co-create and fulfill your true purpose in life, is truly a divine experience. Of course, we can all debate the universal questions such as What is life? Why are we here? and How do I achieve health, happiness, and abundance? Yet I believe that my most meaningful epiphanies and times of peace and blessed assurance have been when I began to perceive my experiences in new ways, which in turn bloomed into liberating feelings of gratitude, happiness, and hope for healing.

So, take off your blinders, hats, and other obstacles that limit your horizons. Instead, embrace the inherent power that you have to co-create the health and the life that you are meant to lead. This book will propel you further than you've ever imagined and explored. It will enable you to make the paradigm shift that can only happen when you invite all of your senses to fully and positively perceive, feel, and believe that the health, peace, and mission you seek can be realized.

PART ONE

Creating True Health

1

Are You Ready for True Health?

Beloved, I pray that all may go well with you and that you may be in good health, just as it is well with your soul.
—3 John 1:2 (New Revised Standard)

Most people come to the Rice Diet Program thinking they want to fix something that is broken. They feel deep in their gut that something is wrong with their bodies and are often afraid of what their further indifference might cause. The majority come to lose weight, then usually within a week of being here they realize that the root of their so-called food problem is really not the food. Their habitual overconsumption of food is instead a physical manifestation, or symptom, of a deeper issue.

Although most Ricers still come to us because of a desire to lose weight, they soon discover that our approach is about far more than looking good. But Lesley was one of those who clearly came on a medical mission. Although she wanted to weigh about a hundred pounds less than her 265 pounds, it was her serious diabetes complications that propelled her to the Rice Diet Program. Lesley had been a diabetic for nearly six years. Like many diabetics, she was more prone to getting infections, and an unattended cold led to her contracting bronchitis, which resulted in a high fever and her developing diabetic ketoacidosis. She landed in the hospital, where she was treated for pneumonia and was instructed to take large amounts of insulin, as well as medications to lower her blood pressure and cholesterol. She knew she had to do something that would stop this potential train wreck, and fast, so she came to the Rice Diet Program.

This is how Lesley describes her experience:

One of the best things I've learned by being on the Rice Diet is that I can have control over my diabetes. Getting off insulin and oral meds has been a huge boost, both physically and emotionally, and it's been encouraging me onward, to continue to exercise and eat better. I realize this *dieta* is my choice, and I can continue my improved health. Taking the time for myself to have a better quality of life, whether it's exercising, going to meals at the Rice House and eventually taking the time to fix healthy meals at home, having a massage, taking a yoga class, or getting together with the important people in my life, I've learned that it's key to take the time for myself, both physically and mentally. Not using food as a source of comfort has been a challenge for me. I'm more aware of the rawness of my stressors, emotions, and feelings sometimes, and I'm searching for different ways of dealing with this. Writing things down has been a help, one way of coping and creating better solutions (instead of creating more problems or accepting the status quo by eating). I've resurrected my journal and frequently write on one of three different blogs. I've also started keeping in better contact with friends and will often pick up the phone or drop someone an e-mail, whether something great has happened and I want to celebrate, or something is troubling me and food is tempting as a coping mechanism. I now enjoy a wider variety of social activities—not just eating!

In addition to losing weight and healing her diabetes, Lesley can boast lowering her blood pressure to 90/60 without any blood pressure medication. Anyone who has practiced the Rice Diet for a while realizes that there is no faster, safer, and more effective way to lose weight and reverse chronic diseases and their risk factors.

Although the reversal of her heart disease risk factors is admirable, what is most exciting and contagious about Lesley's story is that she has taken back her power to co-create the health and the life she desires. Sure, her serious disease states have been healed, but her internal paradigm shift is the most notably profound and pivotal change she has made. It will fuel her healing and enable her to achieve the other life goals she has set for herself.

What our dear Ricers soon learn is that whether you want to lose ten pounds or a hundred pounds, you will not find lasting success if you don't address the deepest core of yourself. And when most people actually look more deeply into themselves, they discover that their problems—whether these are extra weight, disease, emotional issues, or mental stress—are in fact solvable. Indeed, they realize not only that the power to heal is within them, but that they can achieve remarkable health and even newfound joy and passion for life.

So, how do you heal from your inner core? And what is true health? We toss the word *health* around as if we all agree on its meaning or as if there is one static definition of health. Nothing could be further from the truth. Health is not restricted to the body: it involves every aspect of your being—your body, heart, mind, and the most amorphous but most vital part of all—your spirit. The connection between your mental, emotional, and spiritual well-being and your physical health is not only powerful, it's essential, if you truly want to achieve and sustain a life of happiness, enriched by your ability to reach your goals, love the people in your life, and celebrate the very essence of yourself.

Most of us have probably experienced this understanding of our physical, mental, emotional, and spiritual connectedness on some level. Almost everyone has become mentally stressed out or emotionally overwhelmed and then been overcome with a headache or an intense neck ache or back spasm. Although some people may have connected the dots of this cause-and-effect relationship with the various parts of themselves, many "drive on," oblivious of their power to contribute to creating or healing their diseases until it is blatantly obvious—that is, until they are dramatically disabled, ill, or both.

Regardless of why you feel ready for a life change—whether you are motivated by a health crisis, an accident, a divorce, or you simply desire to improve your life and health—you are well on your way to achieving the results you seek. I will show you that you have far more power to create health and reverse disease than you realize. Much of the information you need to attain true health is in your hands!

It's Time to Ask Yourself Some Questions

The Rice Diet Renewal asks a lot of you, but it delivers a lot, too. Take, for example the Ricer whose story follows. He enjoyed significant physical health improvements while on the program, but it was the inner healing that he accomplished that really saved his life. In *The Rice Diet Cookbook*, this doctor shared the medical miracles that he experienced with the Rice *dieta*. When I recently asked him whether he cared to share any deeper emotional and spiritual paradigm shifts that may have accompanied his physical transformations, he again exceeded all of my expectations.

As a doctor, my life prior to my experiences at the Rice Diet Program had been pretty mundane and, worse, had been fairly typical of many of my patients in America. I was rapidly approaching middle age and had been gaining my "obligatory" one to two pounds per year since I was twenty-five. I was about fifty pounds overweight, hypertensive, and losing both my health and my enthusiasm for doing much of anything. I was at the start of what I call the death spiral. I began to feel that life was not worth living anymore, that my only way out was suicide. Fortunately, as a doctor I knew the behavior I was exhibiting by its name—suicidal ideation—and knew that it was an ominous sign that I needed help, and fast.

I thought that the Rice Diet Program was only about food and weight. Although these are important elements, they are only part of the puzzle. The *dieta* represents a way of life, not just a way of eating. The first few weeks were spent in ridding myself of old—and bad—habits related to eating and exercise. I did not realize it at the time, but my spirit was also beginning to heal, through inspiration and interaction with my fellow "Ricers." For the first time in many, many years, I was beginning to value myself as a human being and was gaining insight into further ways to heal both my body and spirit. In a short time at the Rice House, I lost thirty pounds, my blood pressure normalized, and I no longer had diabetic symptoms. I was able to completely discontinue four different types of medications, and I felt better than I had in years.

I am now able to enjoy sports I had not played in twenty-five years. Although most people think I'm crazy, each Saturday you will find me happily jumping out of airplanes, freefalling, and landing under canopy. I remember my father, speaking at our rehearsal dinner the night before our wedding eighteen years ago. He toasted us, with the specific wish that I find some joy in life. Thanks to the Rice Diet Program, I have.

Sincerely, Doc

Meet my friend Doc, whose before and after photos beautifully illustrate his choice to turn his overweight, chronic disease—impaired life into a healthy, active, and exciting one!

When I think about how to achieve true, lasting health, another memorable Ricer comes to mind. Charles, a sixty-year-old veteran twelve-stepper, came to the Rice Diet Program to lose weight and gain control over his health. My journalizing experientials usually begin with a summary of the health benefits and the healing potential of expressive writing. After a brief meditation that facilitates the participants' getting in touch with their deeper thoughts and feelings, I ask the group to write about what came up for them. I encourage them not to try to manufacture something profound but simply to start writing about what comes into their hearts or minds.

I followed the same procedure with Charles's group. After only ten minutes of writing, Charles quietly waited for the others to finish. When the group members were offered time to share their experiences, Charles summarized his life story. He told us that his dad had died when he was very young, and he had to help his mom raise the nine other kids. He was a committed Catholic, who saw to it that his siblings went to church and were educated. As he shared his history, you could feel the spiritual depth of a man who had been forced by

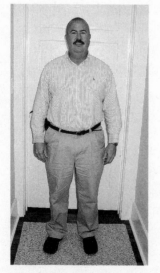

Doc, before starting the Rice Diet Program.

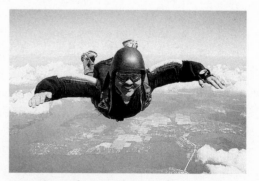

Doc, after embracing the Rice dieta and flourishing with less weight, more health, and a renewed spirit.

circumstances outside of his control to shoulder heavy duties at a much younger age than you would wish on anyone. One of the cards he had been dealt in life was to take on responsibilities for many other people, and his loving and generous spirit was the obvious fruition of this life. He told the group that he was struggling with making a decision about divorce. The burden that such a spiritually mature and sensitive man would feel about this decision, given his caretaker, "hold-the-family-together-at-all-costs" history, melted everyone's heart. To be able to truly speak your truth, with a supportive community that has no agenda, is a profoundly healing opportunity—an experience that enabled Charles to heal in the deepest core of his being and gather the courage to make changes in his life.

Although his heart disease, diabetes, and obesity concerns inspired his initial decision to come to our program, it was his sincere desire to heal his heart at a deeper level that he found most fulfilling and transformative. He was ready to hear his truth; he wrote this poem in only ten minutes!

Sailing from Cape Fear to Hope Island

As I have embarked on this life's journey I simply seem to have just "cast off my dock lines" and headed out to sea. It seems to me today that I have done this without a ship captain's log. But there again I have never really felt like the captain of my ship or the master of my fate.

I am now far out at sea but I can still see land. I remember reading a statement one day that hit me between the eyes. "You can't discover new oceans if you don't leave the sight of land."

I now look to my past life's paths and see that I always seemed to hang on the side of the pool; this was important when I had not yet learned to swim. I can remember asking what the deepest water the instructor had swum in was.

I still remember her answering—like I was still there. "If you learn how to swim, the water depth will have no bearing on your swimming." My fear was not being able to "touch bottom" or to hang on the side. I wanted to be safe. I had no real faith that I could really do this, until I let go and swam.

I am just now learning how to swim in my life stream.

This amazing man was awakening to the desire for wholeness and health. He, like many others, survived his early childhood dramas, unconsciously playing out his pain by co-creating a less-than-fulfilling marriage, and made other mindless choices such as adopting the average American *dieta* of fast foods and other high-saturated-fat and high-sodium foods, inactivity, workaholism, and alcoholism. He, like many people, justified his less-than-desirable lifestyle because he viewed his security and quasi-stable home front to be preferable to the unknown alternative of making a major lifestyle change.

The domino effect of unconscious choices that eventually creates poor health is not what anyone really wants. In the developed, industrialized world, it simply tends to occur when we aren't looking or are not staying mindful of what we are physically doing (eating, exercising, etc.), thinking, feeling, and believing, relative to what we intuitively and passionately want to do with our lives.

Finding the Support You Need

The experiences of Doc and Charles continue to remind me that it doesn't take a lot of time to become honest and consciously connect with ourselves and others, but it does take showing up. If you cannot come to our program at this time, I strongly encourage you to find an emotionally and spiritually supportive community where you are given the opportunity to share and be honest. It doesn't necessarily require a minister, a rabbi, a therapist, or a meditation teacher to facilitate your healing. Many have found a mature 12-step program sponsor

(continued)

to be the only confidential sounding board they needed to recover. Feeling that you are truly *heard* and *known* are important human needs that are often neglected in our fast-paced world. Prioritize the fulfillment of this need; showing up and sharing honestly are important to your health.

It seems that many people feel as if they have superficial acquaintances but few true friends whom they can honestly share everything with. To share your soul and life's challenges with someone who desires to listen and get to know you, without having a vested interest in your specific issue per se, is a healing gift. Two years ago, after a very close girlfriend died of cancer, I prayed for someone to come into my life whom I could share such love and trust with. In less than six months, I met a woman who feels like a sister to me. She started a women's monthly gathering of healing professionals that I now attend. Seek and you will find.

Health emanates when your thoughts, feelings, and beliefs are in alignment with your life choices, and when your actions align with your ideals and convictions. It is your natural state; it is what your body and soul desire to create if you consciously and consistently choose to live with integrity. The opposite of this state would be disease. And while almost everyone would prefer to have good health, this is not to suggest that disease is always a bad thing. In fact, it can be a pivotal and profound teacher, a catalyst for the most revealing experience in your life. Regardless of what the so-called disease looks like or what form it takes (physical, emotional, mental, spiritual, or all four), your first real step toward true health is simply seeing whatever is in your way as a wake-up call prompting you to heal at the root of your symptoms. The more you take inventory of your life, which includes your body, heart, mind, and spirit, the easier it will be for you to see your challenges as learning opportunities to know yourself more deeply, as lessons on your journey toward actualizing your life's purpose.

Your Journal

Although sharing your life, from your diseases to your dreams, can be a powerful part of your healing process, so can writing in general. These are the two main points I emphasize to you now, as I do with all new Rice Diet participants: show up for all program events. For you, reading this now, I encourage you to give your best effort to doing the thirty days of exercises that accompany each level of healing. In fact, I beg you to give them your all. Many times, what you initially judge not to be "your thing" will end up being the experiential that inspires your biggest breakthrough. Some of the techniques may work immediately; others may require a few tries. Certain tools may not resonate with you; others will spark your interest from the get-go. But each step of your journey asks you to "show up" for one or more experientials to engage your body, heart, mind, or spirit. You will have plenty from which to choose, but one of the most important is keeping a journal, in which you will record your experiences—inner and outer, including both feelings and facts.

Your journal can be a three-hole binder with lined paper, a spiral-bound notebook, or a handmade, artful one. Start to document your process; this will help you on your introspective journey and will inspire you to get back on track in three to six months, when you may temporarily lose your way. One of the most powerful ways to get in touch with your thoughts, feelings, beliefs, and life choices is to write them down. Yes, this means you, right now.

Start by answering the following questions in your journal:

Day 1: Inventory of Your Physical, Mental, Emotional, and Spiritual Health Goals

1. When you selected this book, what was your first thought or hope about what you wanted to *heal at the core of your being*?

2. List the top five to ten goals that you would like to co-create in your life in the next five years; be as specific as possible. Take off your blinders and hard hat, think outside your previously held limiting belief system, and boldly write what you really want, need, or have always felt compelled to do.

3. If you have a physical problem or pain that you are ready to reverse, have you ever considered what its underlying emotional root might be? (Hint: Sometimes these are so blatantly obvious that we miss them. Examples could include having a physical "pain in the neck" from dealing with a metaphorical one; my dad had a heart attack after a heart-breaking divorce; many overweight Ricers have told me that weight has served as an insulation.) Describe the thoughts that first came to you.

4. What will your life be like when you achieve your goals? Identify some of the most delightful benefits of actualizing your goals; have fun connecting with the freedom and joy you are imagining.

5. How has this disease or undesired status, situation, or frame of mind served you? What will you give up or lose when you achieve your goal or desired change?

6. Are you ready to manifest your goal? If you are not ready, describe how this present state is serving you; explore your thoughts, feelings, and beliefs on this.

The Scientific Proof for the Benefits of Expressive Writing

Dr. James Pennebaker and Sandra Beall's early research on expressive writing showed that students who journaled about both facts *and* feelings had far fewer visits to the student health center than those who simply journaled about facts *or* feelings. In only four months, the students in the former group enjoyed a 50 percent drop in the monthly visitation rate to the student health center.

(continued)

At our program, Dr. Kitty Klein recently presented a review of twenty years of expressive writing research, showing that people who use expressive writing to convey their thoughts and emotions related to stress and traumatic events enjoy many long-term gains in wellness. In terms of physical benefits, studies have shown that subjects who use the expressive writing technique for self-communication regarding stress or trauma have superior immune function and better general health. Results show both clinical outcomes: improved lymphocyte response, as well as reported outcomes—fewer symptoms, fewer physician visits, and fewer days' stay in the hospital. Psychological effects of expressive writing include better moods, decreased depression, fewer sleep disturbances, and improved working memory. Dr. Klein also explained that in addition to positive health outcomes, writing affects the fundamental cognitive process.

Following are some long-term benefits of expressive writing.

Health Outcomes

- Fewer stress-related visits to the doctor
- Improved immune system functioning
- Reduced blood pressure
- Improved lung function
- Improved liver function
- Fewer days in the hospital
- Improved mood/affect
- A feeling of greater psychological well-being
- Reduced depressive symptoms before examinations
- Fewer post-traumatic intrusion and avoidance symptoms
- Reductions in pain and fatigue and improved psychological well-being in fibromyalgia patients

(continued)

Social and Behavioral Outcomes

- Reduced absenteeism from work
- Quicker reemployment after job loss
- Improved working memory
- Improved sports performance
- Higher grade point average for students
- Altered social and linguistic behavior

People who have the following medical conditions may benefit from participating in expressive writing programs:

- Impaired lung functioning due to asthma
- Disease severity in rheumatoid arthritis
- Pain and deteriorating physical health in cancer
- Immune response in HIV infections
- Hospitalizations for cystic fibrosis
- Pain intensity in women with chronic pelvic pain
- Sleep-onset latency in poor sleepers

"Project Raquel"

Raquel first came to the Rice Diet Program on December 22, 2007. She and her family had left the familiar festivities of their home in the Dominican Republic and decided to spend a healthier Christmas in Durham, North Carolina. Raquel's story dramatically captures the power of expressive writing and journalizing to create health and manifest one's dreams.

My weight was 351 pounds, and my blood pressure was 148/85. Today my weight is 194 pounds and blood pressure is 98/60—and I feel just great. I was not on any medication before, but I am glad that I took control of my life before having to start.

Journalizing is definitely an empowering and rewarding experience; my favorite time to write is before I go to sleep because usually it is a quiet and precious time. My journal is playing an important role in my weight loss and lifestyle change—which I already consider a success. I write about facts and feelings, and this helps me think, explore, understand, and heal. And keeping my journal has helped me change my attitude toward food. I used to eat when happy, sad, stressed . . . now I eat my meals and enjoy every single one. Now I understand and experience things that I once thought were too hard or too silly to try—like being more active, making better food choices, or journalizing. Before going to the Rice Diet Program, I did not cook at all. Now, I cook every time I can, actually enjoy it, and even create my own recipes! The difference is that I have now adopted a healthy lifestyle, and what really matters is the steady long-term results. I truly believe this *dieta* is the answer to all of my years of dieting. Thanks to all the great support from the doctors and the wonderful staff at the Rice Diet Program, this is possible. *I am facing "Project Raquel" with passion, responsibility, and discipline. I set a goal, and I know I will accomplish it.*

Taking Responsibility Is the First Step

In modern industrialized societies, it is rare that anyone is in a place of optimal health. Indeed, most of us are in need of healing— whether from some sort of physical ailment, such as a weight problem, or from a mental impairment, an emotional trauma, a spiritual struggle, or any combination of the above. After many personal and professional experiences with disease, I've started to view all ailments as incredibly similar, while also being unique to each person.

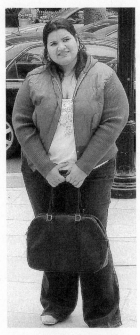
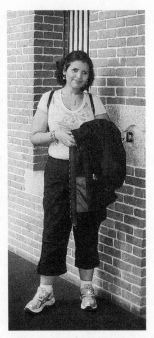

Raquel, before going on the Rice Diet Program.

Raquel, enjoying her journey of "Project Raquel."

Indeed, I know the truth of this because I experienced a very personal awakening to the emotional and spiritual underpinnings of physical disease.

Despite my knowing that mental, emotional, and spiritual issues can create physical disease when left unattended, I apparently needed a wake-up call to understand this more fully in my own life. At that time, I believed that because I followed a semi-vegetarian diet and was a triathlete, I would avoid ill health. But I soon learned just how intimately connected physical health was to my emotional, mental, and spiritual state.

I awoke one New Year's Day crippled from head to toe, which transformed my life in an instant. Although my recovery required nine months of inner healing and included all of the techniques described in the four levels of healing (plus some extras you'll find in chapter 7), the growth, gifts, and rewards I found in this gestational period were worth every ounce of the pain I suffered.

Many facets of my healing experience will be described throughout the book, but at this point I will summarize that this resurrection experience taught me to listen to my inner voice over anyone else's; to really get honest with my words (mind), feelings, and faith; and to require that of my healing team as well.

After a couple of visits with one of the most respected rheumatologists at Duke, the doctor told me to come back next month so that he could watch my progression. I suddenly realized that he did not expect me to recover. I told him that I was interested in watching my regression, not my progression, and that I needed to know whether he thought I would be healed. When he finally admitted that I should get my affairs in order because I would be in a wheelchair within two years, I politely informed him that I would not be in need of his time and that I needed a doctor who believed in healing because I planned on being healed.

As I look back and glean the components that were pivotal to my tenacious pursuit and successful realization of healing, I believe the following ones to be essential:

- My readiness, desire, and will to be free from pain and disability was enormous.
- My mind was informed about the issue (I read every mind, body, and spirit book I could find).
- I felt hopeful, which fueled my expectancy and tenacity.
- I truly believed that I would be totally healed.
- My faith in God deepened, and faith moves God. (If you do not believe in God, you may prefer substituting the words "the natural, creative source of power," which can facilitate shifts in energy and co-create your healing.)

It was a terrifying, painful, and humbling nine-month experience that, in retrospect, was one of the best things that ever happened to me. Through the fear, pain, and self-examination of that time, I learned how to dig deeply into what actually had crippled me and take responsibility for the emotions that I had unconsciously allowed to preoccupy my thoughts, dreams, and energy (even on a cellular and subatomic level). I sought a total healing from the Creative source that is within us all. After I fired the supposed "best rheumatologist at Duke," I sought the opinion of an allergist, because I had concurrently contracted serious allergies. (I knew that arthritis and allergies were both autoimmune diseases, a symptom that my body was turning against itself, and I sensed that their timing was not a coincidence.)

After the new doctor questioned me about my *dieta* for forty minutes, I thanked him for his thorough assessment and reminded him that I wanted to know what he knew about the allergy-arthritis connection. He turned to his prescription pad and wrote his order: "Count squirrels on the Eno River 2 hours/day."

And then, with great wisdom, he stated, "Ms. Gurkin, you do not have arthritis; you have a stress-induced joint condition that you can heal if you do what you are telling your heart patients to do!"

The longer I processed and examined my pain, via journalizing, meditation, and prayer, the more clearly I realized that I had crippled myself through my own unresolved habitual tendency to be resentful of controlling people. Specifically, in the face of any authority figure who did not respect my opinion, I would respond with anger, turning these strident feelings inward.

What I would discover through my own healing journey was that when I finally became *ready* to release my false belief that I was the authority of anything and thus could let go of my resentment of others, I would be free of certain deeply ingrained habits of body, mind, and spirit that had caused my joints to rebel and seize up. (Some people would call this an example of healing a control addiction.)

Being *ready* does not mean we will be healed instantly, but it does fuel our tenacity, hope, and belief that all will be well if we persevere and keep our eyes on the prize. Through each chapter's lens, you will become more and more ready and able to take full responsibility for what your body is telling you, then for what your mind, heart, and spirit are communicating at subtler levels. As you cleanse your body with optimal whole organic foods and exercise, it will become ever easier to hear from each of your aspects and to really trust your own truth. By actually participating in the process and actively

responding to the challenges put forth within this book, you will experience an openness and a willingness that are subtle, yet essential,
for healing at the core. Although other people's epiphanies are
inspiring, you need to participate firsthand to get the results you
most want—which are your own. This is not a spectator sport!

When you choose to believe that you are responsible for your
health, you gain a sense of empowerment and control. The following Ricer Forum story, from someone who has lost seventy pounds
and has won an immeasurable amount of self-knowledge and inner
peace, captures the essence of this positive domino effect:

> For me, the Rice Diet has meant empowerment. I didn't
> realize until I had started the program and cleansed my
> body—and spirit—that I had lived *my entire life* powerless
> to others. I allowed their emotions to control mine, then
> I ate through mine because I didn't want to cause someone
> else pain. I had to be the "happy one," but when I wasn't, the
> only way I knew to become happy was to find consolation in
> food, which I did—almost hourly some days.
>
> I had become a puppet in my own life, waiting for the
> next event to happen, but not making it happen myself. I had
> never learned to be in the moment and to enjoy life, because
> all I had ever learned to enjoy was food, and there is only so
> much "good" food out there, isn't there?
>
> For the last year, I've kept off seventy pounds and feel more
> in control of who I am, as well as my eating, than I have ever
> been in my life. I have had numerous "events" and emotional
> setbacks this year, but I have not given in—or given up. The
> calm of a clean and healthy *dieta* supports me through these
> events, giving me a sense of empowerment I have never felt
> before. While I have not eaten "perfect" every moment, I ate
> those things with mindfulness. If I am going to eat chocolate
> or a dessert, I am going to do so and enjoy it, knowing I am no
> longer chained to eating this way daily. I have become so "in
> tune" with my body that when I do eat something outside of the
> *dieta*, I almost immediately feel bloated, light-headed, or just

downright irritable. How great is that?! I have learned that my body wants to be healthy. I feel like I can control my emotions and my life now, through the support of this healthy lifestyle.

As most of you know, amazing feats and incredible accomplishments do not fall out of the sky onto your head. Greatness and success have long been correlated with knowing who you are and what you want, connecting with that passion and purpose, and then undertaking lots of practice, practice, practice. It has repeatedly been shown that ten thousand hours of practice are required before any of the greatest musicians, athletes, artists, or actors achieved their star status: they made a conscious decision, established their goals, created a plan to reach those goals, and then practiced, practiced, and practiced. They achieved their dreams because they lived their dreams every day. And yet studies show that less than 1 percent of Americans actually write down their specific goals each year. This is really a tragic loss of potential.

So, right now, take a moment to imagine a goal that has always seemed beyond your reach. Think big; choose something you really want, even if at first it seems unobtainable—such as your ideal body weight, to be a nonsmoker, to be in a loving, supportive relationship. Co-creating true health will require your getting clear about what you want for your body, mind, heart, and spirit and delving deeper into the ways to obtain it. First, think about what you want, imagine what that will feel like when you co-create or attract it, and believe that it is yours to enjoy.

Day 2: Develop Your Dream Board

Have you written down what you are seeking to create in your life? Even after my encouragement, your honest answer may still be no. Well, in this present moment you can choose to actually show up and participate in co-creating the health and the life you want. Get your notebook, your journal, or at least a piece of paper. You now can begin to articulate and then write down your goals, with specific plans to achieve them. After specifying your goals in black and white, you may be amazed at what a difference it can make to take it to the next level in Technicolor and add your sense of touch. A tactile experiential brings a whole new dimension of sensation into the paradigm-shifting equation. As you will appreciate more later, while you do this Dream Board project, your brain is laying down more neuronal anchors for these goals and dreams, to enhance your probabilities of achieving success. You can cut out magazine images or collect nature objects to reflect a goal to go on more nature walks or vacations, or anything that reminds you of your desired goals or dreams. Then select a poster board or colorful construction paper to use as the background or base on which you will arrange the objects. Use a glue stick or attach them to your poster board somehow. Your imagination is the limit to how creative and liberating this exercise will be. I have seen participants frame and texturize their creations with incredibly beautiful finds from their Eno River hikes, which prompts them to remember how restorative nature and other Rice Diet/Durham experiences were for them. Others made 3D creations, such as cutting out an incredibly ornate window so that it actually opened into a dream vacation spot. Another person tied a CD onto the board in the center to reinforce her dream of finally cutting her first musical CD. The Dream Board assignment may take you a few days to prepare just the right images or objects for your upcoming vision or goal statement, so feel free to write your goals today, complete with detailed plans on how to enact them. Then set an appointment for yourself or with a friend within the next week to complete your artistic rendition.

Although this Dream Board assignment may at first sound like a Girl Scout project or a senior citizen center's afternoon entertainment that you perceive to be beneath you or too much trouble because of your busy schedule, think again. This experiential is one of the more enjoyable and enlightening art forms I have witnessed. One day last year, Kate, a fellow Ricer who always showed up for classes, came to the Dream Board session. She was ready, willing, and open to the new, multisensory experiential:

> Today I made a Dream Board with Kitty Rosati. I cut out pictures
> from magazines that represented my goals and dreams for the

next one to five years. It was easy to find a lot of pictures that "spoke to me" of my dream life. As I was thinking about how I wanted to display my pictures, it hit me—I am looking at my life as it is now! I already have my dream life! And I didn't even know it! I already have everything that I cut out to illustrate my dream life, . . . I just don't "show up" for it! I already have a beautiful garden, but I stay inside because I feel too overweight to be seen outside tending it. I already have a loving husband and son to scuba dive with on vacations, yet due to my lack of acceptance of my body, I stay in the hotel room while they explore exotic South Pacific reefs. I suddenly realized that I am so unhappy with my weight that I shut myself out from my life, and I wouldn't allow myself to enjoy anything until I lost the weight. But I've decided to enjoy my own party, to "show up for the dream life I already have" instead of thinking I have to be thinner to do so. I don't want to waste any more time! If I hadn't done this Dream Board, I may not have ever realized what I already have! I am even more determined to get this weight off now, so I can live my dreams with health and longevity.

When Kate shared this epiphany with us, her eyes were filled with tears, and everyone present knew that we were standing with her on hallowed ground. That much truth, when experienced from a deep place, is palpable, and her readiness and desire for healing spread to others.

The upcoming chapters will guide you to clarify your plan to achieve this and other goals. The four levels of healing that make up the Rice Diet Renewal program are so powerful, they not only offer everyone a path to lose weight and heal disease, but they also provide methods to help you access your true self and accomplish your biggest, most important goals.

The real meaning of health is when the body, mind, heart, and spirit awaken and connect to create and express a person's fullest potential. When you achieve true health, your dreams, goals, and extraordinary desires become not only possible but probable. That is the ultimate promise of *The Rice Diet Renewal*.

2

Cleansing Your Body

*Nothing will benefit human health and increase chances
for survival of life on Earth as much as the evolution to a
vegetarian diet.*
—Albert Einstein

Remember the old axiom "If you don't have your health, you don't have anything"? Therein lies a great truth. "Cleansing Your Body" is the beginning of your journey. This chapter focuses on the physical realm: your body. Often, it is easiest for people to identify with their bodies, to clarify what is wrong physically and what they must change, and to recognize the beneficial results that come from following healthy guidelines. When you lose unwanted weight and cleanse your body of toxins that have accumulated from a diet of processed foods laden with excess sodium, fat, and sugar, you will begin to taste and smell again. When you feel lighter, start to think more clearly, and experience an optimistic outlook on life, then you are in a much better position to be inspired to seek deeper realms of healing that will support and sustain your journey toward true health.

Many people come to the Rice Diet Program because they are ready to feel better; most of them also want to lose weight. Inevitably, they have read or heard of the Rice Diet Program's incredible results. Since 1939, participants have lost unwanted pounds faster, and more safely, and have maintained their weight loss longer, than with any other diet program ever documented. Men lose an average of thirty pounds each and women an average of nineteen pounds in the first month on the program. Furthermore, 43 percent of Ricers maintain their weight loss or lose even more after six years! Their desire to feel and look better is often preceded by a growing concern for their risk of developing heart disease, obesity, high blood pressure, high cholesterol, or diabetes. Sometimes they become motivated to change after undergoing a near-death experience such as a heart attack or a personal trauma—perhaps a divorce or the death of a loved one. Other times, people simply want to change the way they have been eating and living because they experience an overwhelming sense of discontent, knowing that they need to make a major change in their lives, or else.

The Rice Diet Program has always focused on promoting good health and on preventing and reversing disease. The optimal health that we seek is not merely an absence of disease; it is a vibrancy and an aliveness that results from eating clean whole foods, engaging in regular exercise, and taking time to reclaim the power that is within us. Although most of us have taken a few undesirable detours or painful shortcuts on our journey through life, our return to vibrant health and happiness depends on our realizing that we have the ability to resurrect ourselves, to reconnect with our power and passionately pursue our gifts and intentions. It is crucial to take this first step toward physical healing as if your life and your health really matter. Remember that even though diet and exercise are the focus of this chapter and will initially produce the most obvious results, the fruition of your good health will be rooted in the awareness and belief that you are able: the Latin meaning of *power* is "to be able."

To begin this journey, let's first focus on your body. What is your main goal? Do you want to lose weight, stabilize your blood sugar, or heal a certain disease? By first connecting with how your body feels and functions, you are one step closer to manifesting the optimal health that you desire.

I recommend cleaning up your diet first—and not only because I have a master's degree in foods and nutrition. I think that an organic, whole-food diet without added sodium will improve your physical health, as well as your thoughts, feelings, and spiritual openness to the creative process, faster than any other concrete thing you can do for yourself. One of the main ways that the Rice Diet cleanses your body of toxins, excess pounds, and other impurities is through its low-sodium nature.

The Skinny on Sodium

Since its inception in 1939, the Rice Diet has been defined as a medical therapy based on a "no-salt-added diet." Dr. Walter Kempner founded the Rice Diet Program to treat hypertensives and kidney patients. At that point in history, there were no blood pressure–lowering medications or dialysis machines available; thus, patients with very high blood pressure (malignant hypertensives) and kidney disease either followed the Rice Diet or died before the age of forty. Seventy years of Rice Diet experience have shown that significantly reducing our sodium intake can dramatically improve or heal a wide range of health conditions that conventional medicine often fails to alleviate. Miracles upon miracles are documented on our walls and in our files, from malignant hypertensives who normalized their blood pressure, to those blinded (legally confirmed blind) from previously uncontrolled diabetes who regained their vision and left driving newly needed cars!

During the last two decades, I have personally observed, and research has documented, a growing concern for the deleterious effects of sodium consumption on our health. Globally speaking, cardiovascular disease is the leading cause of death and disability, and high blood pressure is the most important contributing factor (accounting for 62 percent of strokes and 49 percent of coronary heart disease).

While there is no doubt that we need to reduce our sodium intake, there is no agreement as to by how much. The current (as of 2005) Dietary Guidelines recommend no more than 2,300 mg of sodium per day for healthy Americans and no more than 1,500 mg for those with hypertension and other sodium sensitivities, African Americans, and people fifty and older. It is reported that one in three U.S. adults—an estimated 73.6 million people—has high blood pressure or hypertension, and an additional 25 to 37 percent of Americans have prehypertension. As reported in *Morbidity and Mortality Weekly Report* in March 2009, this equates to 69 percent of the population being at an increased risk for heart disease and stroke due to having elevated blood pressure.

Since the daily 1,500-mg sodium restriction applies to the majority of the population, the American Heart Association and the American Stroke Association recommend that the 1,500-mg limit apply to the *entire* U.S. population and be reflected in future federal guidelines. Although there has been a call to food manufacturers and restaurants to reduce the amount of salt added to foods by 50 percent over the next ten years, sodium intake in the United States remains high. On the other hand, Great Britain has succeeded in making multinational giants like McDonald's and Kraft use less salt in the foods they produce. But considering our country's track record with enforcing lower-sodium foods from manufacturers and restaurants, and the fact that 77 percent of the sodium in our diet comes from processed foods and restaurant meals, those who want to be healthy must take responsibility for it.

Not only is there very strong evidence that our current consumption of salt is the main factor in elevating our blood pressure and increasing our risk of developing heart disease, strokes, and kidney disease, there is also growing evidence for its correlation with diabetes, obesity, osteoporosis, and stomach cancer. An Australian study showed that when research participants consumed four test meals randomly—equal caloric amounts of brown lentils or white bread, either salted (containing approximately one-third the daily sodium intake of Americans) or unsalted—the concentrations of glucose and plasma insulin were substantially higher in the sub-jects after they consumed the salted meals. In fact, the results were very significant. Forty-five minutes after participants ate the salted lentils, the study reported plasma insulin concentrations to be 22 percent higher than the insulin levels of people who had just eaten the unsalted lentils. Even more dramatic was the difference in insulin concentration after subjects ate salted versus unsalted bread: an average of 39 percent greater during the three hours fol-lowing the meals! Because obesity, high blood glucose (diabetes), and accompanying elevated levels of plasma insulin are considered to be risks for heart disease, why would we want to add salt to our food? More blood sugar in the blood, with more insulin available to take into our cells, does not help us lose weight, and we know that obesity can contribute to all of the modifiable risk factors of heart disease.

Although the absence of added sodium in the Rice Diet was not originally intended for weight-loss purposes, it will not take you long to appreciate its importance. There is no wake-up call more powerful for an overeater than a no-salt-added whole-food plan; the obsessive thoughts and overeating tendencies are usually silenced within one to two days. In my two decades of coaching Ricers, I've observed their amazement at the dramatic reduction of their appetite and food obsessions. This has been the most memorable and life-altering aspect of the diet. Interestingly enough, the more overweight a person is, the more dramatic his or her surprise at the cessation of previous food fixations. One man described it to me as feeling like he had been "let out of jail from a place where his brain had felt possessed by the unrelenting calls from food."

We all know that salt and other sodium-containing ingredi-ents are flavor enhancers, thus making us want to eat more, but no one yet fully understands how high sodium intake can lead to obesity. An interesting article in the September 2007 issue of *Obesity* reported that rats that ate a high-salt diet had increased white adipose mass, meaning an increase in the size and number of fat cells, when compared to rats that ate normal and low-salt diets. In addition, the rats on the high-salt diet ate more and had higher blood pressure than did the rats on the low-salt diet. While we humans are more evolved than rats, we certainly should be taking some notes here!

Although many large health organizations in the United States publish reports that call for a major reduction in the salt content of processed and restaurant foods, little real change has actually been implemented. For the food industry to change, we must change; vote with your dollars and don't buy processed foods. Long term, you will save more money than you can count. When people tell me that they can't afford to buy whole foods, my usual response is "Pay now, or you and your children will pay later!"

There are also hidden costs that result from having a diet of processed foods: first, medical bills due to health problems caused by consuming this high-sodium, low-fiber, nutrient-inferior food; and second, the environmental and ethical problems that many people are unconsciously creating by supporting conventionally grown, highly processed, and transported foods. More on this later.

The Rice Diet Simplified

The Rice Diet is made up of whole grains, beans, fruits, and vegetables that are free of processed ingredients; the diet is naturally low in fat and sodium and has a minor emphasis on seafood and other low-saturated-fat animal products (if they are appropriate for one's health). The importance of avoiding refined, highly addictive foods that are rich in sugar, salt, and fat (especially saturated or trans fats) cannot be overemphasized. These are triggers for people who struggle with overeating and obesity, and they correlate strongly with an increased risk of developing most chronic diseases (heart disease and its risk factors, cancer, arthritis, etc.). Although part of me hesitates to say *avoid*, because I don't want to set you up for feeling deprived, I must repeat the twelve-step advice: "If you don't want to fall down, don't go onto slippery places!" If healing is really a priority for you, you can avoid these slippery places for at least a month, which is how much time you'll need to give yourself to absorb this new dietary information, cleanse your palate, and enjoy the progress you are making. There is nothing quite as inspiring as palpable improvements and dramatic results to motivate you to keep going!

For those of you who have read my books, *Heal Your Heart, The Rice Diet Solution*, and/or *The Rice Diet Cookbook*, you will notice that this description of the diet is condensed. If you would like more detailed specifics about the diet, such as portion sizes and the nutritional averages of various food groups, you may consult any of these books for a refresher course and to peruse their bounty of delicious recipes and menus. You can also find this detailed information about food groups and portion sizes extracted for you from the *Journal for Health* booklet that is offered on our Web site (www.ricediet.com). The essence and power of the diet can easily by achieved without your counting a calorie, a gram of fat, or a milligram of sodium, but people who want more nutritional details can refer to the upcoming menus' specific recipes (in the back of this book), complete with nutritional analyses.

For newbies in the group, rest assured that this general description and four weeks of menus will produce the same results!

The diet is built around your eating a total of 1,000 calories per day and asks that you exercise at least one hour each day. Obviously, people who are unable to exercise this much immediately need to gradually increase their activity, depending on their doctor's recommendation. If you follow this regimen, you will lose weight as fast and effectively as you desire. Although the first month of weight loss is phenomenal, with men averaging a pound a day and women losing more than half a pound a day, this rate will slow down as you get closer to your goal. The good news is that even those of us with only ten pounds or so to lose can continue to enjoy one to two pounds of weight loss per week.

Just keep your food intake simple. Eat whole foods that look like they did when they were harvested. Avoid products that contain ingredients with added sodium and animal fats or partially hydrogenated fats, and buy organic whenever possible. Remember, the lower your intake of sodium, sugar, and processed, refined ingredients, the less will be your appetite and desire to overeat.

For people who find that they still desire more than the 1,000 recommended calories, rest assured that even if you increase your intake to 1,200 or 1,500 calories, you will still lose weight; the process will simply be slower. Just be sure that the foods you consume are whole, unprocessed foods, without salt, sugar, or refined ingredients. If you follow these guidelines with awareness, assisted by this book's inner healing guidance, you will achieve and maintain your health and weight goals.

The Rice Diet's plan for home use has been divided into three phases in my previous two books. Although that has proved helpful for thousands of readers, the following description will simplify this process and enable the reader to focus on what is most important: eating whole foods, unsalted and unprocessed. Inherent in this very basic and simple approach is allowing yourself plenty of time to heal at your core. You will investigate your previous history and beliefs about food by applying fresh knowledge and attention to the underlying reasons that you have not previously practiced an optimally healthy *dieta*, and you will map your game plan to successfully do so now.

Why the Rice Diet Works

- It is a detox diet that cleanses your body, ridding it of excess sodium, water weight, and many toxins from processed foods and the environment. Once your palate and body are cleansed and returned to a natural state, most people find that they begin to prefer healthy, unprocessed foods.

- It is a low-sodium diet that limits salt and all other sodium-rich ingredients to 500–1,000 mg daily. Salt, like sugar, stimulates your appetite. When sodium is not added to your diet, you rid yourself of a powerful appetite stimulant

(continued)

and get in touch with your natural ability to taste and enjoy moderate portions of whole foods. You actually become conscious of what you are consuming. As a result, you innately control your eating behavior; your eating behavior does not control you.

- It is a low-fat diet that especially limits saturated fats. While it is true that the lower your fat intake, the lower your weight and the better your odds for maintaining your desired weight, the most important fat to limit is saturated fat, which comes primarily from animal fats. Keep in mind, however, that some fats are health-promoting and therefore good for you to eat, such as olive oil, walnuts, sesame seeds, flaxseeds, and fish. By avoiding corn-fed animal products and enjoying only organic and free-range (grass-fed) animal products, you will greatly improve your omega-6 to omega-3 fatty acid ratio and reduce your cancer and heart disease risks.

- It is a diet that relies on complex carbohydrates such as grains, beans, veggies, and fruit—all of which are high in fiber that cleanses the body and fills you up. This "whole foods" diet is rich and varied in taste, texture, and nutrients. You no longer crave foods, and you never (or rarely) feel hungry. Slow-absorbing, soluble fiber–rich foods allow everyone, including diabetics and hypoglycemics, to eat complex carbohydrates with confidence and gratitude. Consuming soluble fiber–rich foods, such as oats, beans, and barley, will lower your cholesterol, stabilize your blood sugar, and thus help you feel more full faster.

- It is a diet that is individualized to you. By keeping a food record, you will become more mindful of what you are eating and be aware of which dietary additions (if any) cause a deleterious health response. Otherwise, the diet includes whatever foods that produce the results you desire.

In essence, you will be asked to eat clean, unprocessed, whole foods, simply and mindfully; it is indeed that easy. This is not magic, although the results may often inspire you to feel as if it is. Rather, it is common sense. If the menus later in this chapter do not include your favorite healthy food choices, replace them with your preferences; personalize these menus until they entice you.

You may note that these menus are sensitive to the practical challenges that the average working person might face. Many people take their lunch to work, and leftovers are more practical than preparing a meal from scratch. Sushi rice is loaded with salt and sugar, so I request that my sushi be made with plain steamed rice. After I add wasabi, which contains no added sodium, and a little pickled ginger to each bite, I've created a delicious meal that is full of flavor. It is also easy to eat in a Chinese restaurant by ordering stir-fried vegetables and tofu over steamed rice and requesting that your food be stir-fried in sake (rather than in oil) with extra fresh garlic and ginger; no salt, MSG, or soy sauce. I also ask for fresh lemon wedges and red pepper flakes on the side, to jazz up my dish as I desire. Yum! Be sure to check out our Web site for additional recipes, valuable free support, and more: www.ricediet.com.

Day 3: The Quick-and-Easy Guide

How you follow the diet is up to you. But do keep in mind some advice we have heard over and over again from Ricers themselves: if you really want to lose weight and keep it off, then don't skip meals—eat breakfast, lunch, and dinner. In fact, if you'd like to eat smaller, more frequent meals or snacks in addition to three meals, that's fine, too—just keep up with the day's tally of servings.

The health-promoting pyramid (see the next page) is a good general guide. Jot down your intake of the food group totals in a journal on a daily basis as a powerful mindfulness exercise. Don't get obsessed or overly distracted by fractions of food groups that you eat. Instead, choose suggested servings from the lower end of the range if you are a smaller woman and from the higher end if you are a larger man or someone approaching his or her goal weight or maintenance phase. Note that the calcium-rich foods are highlighted, to assist you in choosing four to six servings of calcium-rich foods each day. If you don't care for these calcium-rich foods, you may prefer to supplement with 1,000 mg of calcium per day.

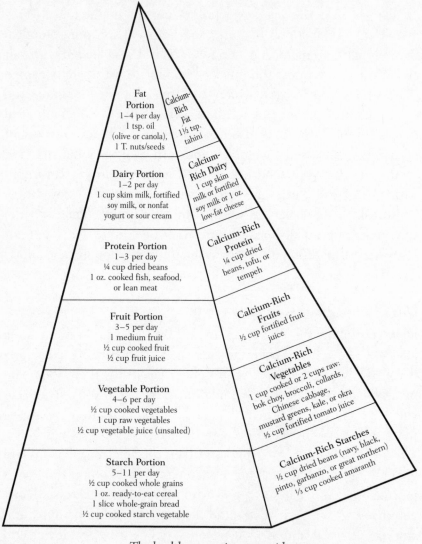

Fat Portion
1–4 per day
1 tsp. oil
(olive or canola),
1 T. nuts/seeds

Calcium-Rich Fat
1½ tsp. tahini

Dairy Portion
1–2 per day
1 cup skim milk, fortified soy milk, or nonfat yogurt or sour cream

Calcium-Rich Dairy
1 cup skim milk or fortified soy milk or 1 oz. low-fat cheese

Protein Portion
1–3 per day
¼ cup dried beans
1 oz. cooked fish, seafood, or lean meat

Calcium-Rich Protein
¼ cup dried beans, tofu, or tempeh

Fruit Portion
3–5 per day
1 medium fruit
½ cup cooked fruit
½ cup fruit juice

Calcium-Rich Fruits
½ cup fortified fruit juice

Vegetable Portion
4–6 per day
½ cup cooked vegetables
1 cup raw vegetables
½ cup vegetable juice (unsalted)

Calcium-Rich Vegetables
1 cup cooked or 2 cups raw: bok choy, broccoli, collards, Chinese cabbage, mustard greens, kale, or okra
½ cup fortified tomato juice

Starch Portion
5–11 per day
½ cup cooked whole grains
1 oz. ready-to-eat cereal
1 slice whole-grain bread
½ cup cooked starch vegetable

Calcium-Rich Starches
½ cup dried beans (navy, black, pinto, garbanzo, or great northern)
⅓ cup cooked amaranth

The health-promoting pyramid.

Daily Food Group Guidelines

Here are the food group guidelines that will help you make your daily food choices. Obviously, eating on the lower end of the range will inspire faster weight loss.

- 4–6 vegetable servings
- 3–5 fruit servings
- 5–11 starch servings
- 1–4 teaspoons of olive oil (or other acceptable fat)
- 1–2 cups of nonfat dairy (or calcium-fortified soy) products
- 1–3 ounces of animal protein or ¼–¾ cup servings of beans

Tips for the Rice Diet

Once-a-Week Detox: The Basic Rice Diet

The Basic Rice Diet is the ultimate detox diet. It has only nutrient-dense whole grains and fruits and contains no salt, refined sugar, or other highly processed triggers that are found in processed foods; if it's organic, it will also be free of preservatives, hormones, antibiotics, and genetically modified organisms. The Basic Rice Diet has the advantages of a fast; it immediately and dramatically reduces your appetite and almost miraculously shifts your food-focused mental processing to be one of mindfulness with life in general. Headaches, insomnia, psoriasis, and many other problems are usually alleviated or drastically reduced within days.

Because most people in industrialized nations eat such a processed conglomerate of natural and artificial ingredients, it is nearly impossible to determine which substances in their diet or environment are causing their problems. Although there are various ways to assess food allergies, the best method is to simplify your intake to foods that are rarely known to cause allergies, then introduce one new food at a time per day and take note. Because the most common foods that are thought to cause allergies include peanuts, dairy, wheat, corn, eggs, and soybeans, the Rice Diet is a great opportunity to identify and eliminate your problem food, if allergies are an issue for you. From this list of foods most likely to cause allergies, only wheat and corn are served at the Rice Diet Program. Therefore, it is quite simple not to select the grits, the shredded wheat, the pasta, or the cream of wheat, and if the allergic response you thought was due to wheat or corn goes away, you may decide that these grains are not worth the side effects you experienced.

Although the Basic Rice Diet is not recommended for more than one day per week, unless you are medically supervised here on the program, the Vegetarian Plus Dairy (or rice or soy dairy substitutes) days are recommended for as long as you like, with a daily multivitamin/mineral and calcium supplement, for great detox results. In previous books I detailed how animal proteins, in addition to the dairy serving, should be limited to three ounces per week until a person reaches his or her ideal body weight. I'm now inviting you to consciously take responsibility for co-creating your own health and life, starting with your dietary choices. Coach Foster, my beloved high school math teacher, often said to me, "Gurkin [my maiden name], read the clues!" He, of course, would say that to anyone not paying attention. So I will pay it forward and invite you to read your clues!

We highly recommend that you follow the Basic Rice Diet *only one day per week*, to safely enjoy the results of the Rice Diet at home. Although the Basic Rice Diet is a powerful detox experience because it is optimally and naturally nutrient-dense and fiber-rich, and includes no trigger ingredients such as sodium, refined foods, and sugar, it is too low in sodium to safely follow for more than one day per week without our medical supervision. But it is well worth the discipline for you to experience this regenerative and enlightening day, because it almost instantly gives you a heightened awareness of the answers to certain essential questions about when, where, and why you habitually turn to food to squelch your stress and undesirable emotions.

Detox! Testimony for a Weekly Basic Rice Diet Day

Last year at the Rice House, a gorgeous, thirty-something Ricer waltzed into the dining room just as everyone was sitting down for lunch. I did a double take before recognizing the woman as someone who had lost yet another thirty pounds since leaving the Rice House. When I ran to hug her and congratulate her on the additional weight loss, I asked her what was the most important advice she could share with others who were pursuing a long-term weight-loss goal.

She did not hesitate before answering: "The most significant difference the Rice Diet has made in my life, which is reflected in my successful weight loss, is my enhanced awareness, and the detox day was a key tool for reinforcing and reclaiming my awareness!"

Her passionate enthusiasm for the detox stage was a convincing confirmation that the Basic Rice Diet day was a worthy practice to institute weekly. Like the many other practices offered here, the Basic Rice Diet day can greatly influence participants to remain aware on so many levels. This woman gladly inspired everyone present with her incredible testimony about how the once-a-week detox day had been instrumental in empowering her long-term weight-loss success by intensely renewing and heightening her awareness.

Protein

The remaining days of the week you will enjoy grains (primarily whole and unprocessed), fruits, vegetables, beans, and dairy or soy products. If you like fish, you can also have three ounces of cooked fish a couple of days per week. Other seafood and occasional eggs and lean meats are fine if you do not have heart disease. If you have a strong family history of heart disease or cancer, limiting animal products is the most proactive preventive measure you can take, next to not smoking cigarettes. Again, realize that you are worth the cost and effort of obtaining the best organic, grass-fed, or free-range animal products available. You really are what you eat, and you usually get what you pay for. More is not better; in fact, consuming less animal products but those of higher quality (if you desire any) is healthier for you and illustrates conscious consumption with an integrity of purpose—for yourself, your fellow animals, your neighbors, farm workers, the natural resources, and the planet.

Dr. Colin Campbell, the author of the world-renowned *The China Study*, suggests that excessive amounts of animal protein predict heart disease more than does fat intake. So if you are still remembering your mother's words when she proudly served and encouraged you to eat your meat, you need to realize that she was doing the best she could with the information she was given. She was likely convinced that meat, which her parents probably could not often afford, was a special and desirable high-protein food. Yet the majority of the world's healthiest and longest-lived people are vegetarians or eat very few animal products (see the sidebar on page 47).

Much of my graduate school nutrition training has been challenged and altered by the real-life results I've witnessed. Dietitians are taught that the human body needs a high-protein diet to heal burns and skin problems or to aid in postsurgery recovery; however, Duke surgeons repeatedly tell us that Ricers have the best postoperative experiences of all the patients they see. I have witnessed skin lesions heal faster than I could believe in a Ricer whose legs had not had healthy skin in years. You may also hear the oft-repeated myth that you need to eat more protein if you want to do strength training. This is not true. One of our young athletic men lost a total of 103 pounds in 161 days, while his strength and endurance improved considerably. His ability to bench press increased from 285 to 370 pounds after he lost the weight. In short, inadequate protein will not be your problem.

So, get ready to assure your less-than-informed, well-intentioned critics that you will get more than enough protein by eating grains, beans, vegetables, and soy milk or low-fat dairy daily.

Specifically, this diet provides sufficient protein via:

- 2–4 cups of cooked grains and/or beans
- 2–6 cups of vegetables
- 1–2 cups of organic dairy or soy milk six days per week

Healing yourself and transforming your perceptions about food, as well as changing how you respond to others' judgments and opinions, are important aspects of developing mindfulness and confidence about your food choices. As you follow the Rice Diet, be mindful of your results. The fruition of this monthlong commitment will convince you, if I haven't.

The Healthiest and Longest-Lived People in the World Eat Simply

Epidemiological research, or studies from various populations around the world, has provided proof for years that a diet that promotes health and longevity doesn't have to be laden with complicated formulas, expensive concoctions, or mysterious secret ingredients from distant lands. In fact, *The Blue Zones: Lessons for Living Longer from the People Who've Lived the Longest*, by Dan Buettner, describes the inverse to be true. The populations in the four areas of the world he investigated had longevity, strength, vitality, and happiness without consulting any dietary experts or following any rigid prescriptive formulas. The diets were inexpensive, homegrown, and basic. From the Nicoyan Peninsula in Costa Rica to Sardinia; to Loma Linda, California; to Okinawa, Japan, the longest-lived people ate very similarly: all had primarily plant-based diets (thus low in saturated fats) and ate mainly handmade foods (consequently, these were naturally low in sodium, saturated fats, and refined carbohydrates). If they ate animal products

(continued)

at all, they consumed fish or grass-fed sheep's cheese (which is naturally rich in omega-3 fatty acids). Like participants of the Rice Diet, these centenarians were not only eating the most optimal, healthiest diet; in general, they exercised daily and focused on their families, friends, and faith. Other lifestyle habits that were cited included eating big breakfasts and smaller meals later in the day, not overeating, prioritizing their ties with the community, and enjoying a strong sense of purpose. Because *The Rice Diet Renewal* will emphasize how to develop a strong foundational support, you will not need to be distracted by dietary details. In fact, you'll be investing your time and focus in arenas that will anchor and enhance your long-term success.

Ensure that you eat a daily serving of dairy and/or soy products and regular cereal or bread serving (which each typically contains more than 100 mg of sodium) to keep your sodium intake sufficient. The only time we've seen people need more sodium than this is if they are running near-marathon distances in humid, ninety-degree weather and are sweating profusely. If this is your lifestyle choice, you may need to drink more than the recommended six to nine 8-ounce glasses of water (or fluids) per day that most of us require, as well as take a couple hundred more milligrams of sodium. You should never "force fluids" or drink excessively on a low-sodium diet.

Sample Menus for the Rice Diet

Check with your medical doctor before starting this or any diet, especially if you are taking medications.

Starting on page 50 is a chart of four sample 1,000-calorie-a-day weekly menus. Monday is designated as the Basic Rice Diet and is 800 calories; it will reinspire and renew your focus and appreciation for whole foods and also remind you of how good the vegetables will be tomorrow! You will also notice that the other days include a dairy or soy milk choice (officially called the Lacto-Vegetarian Rice Diet); and after the first week you may include seafood or other lean, healthfully raised animal products (officially the Vegetarian Plus Rice Diet) if appropriate for your health issues. Please realize that these menus are provided as an example of a health-promoting monthly food plan, not a rigid, required prescription. Personalize these menus to complement your lifestyle and what is doable for you.

As long as your actual daily calorie totals are within 100 calories of either the 1,000-calorie or the 800-calorie maximum, you will see very impressive results from the Rice Diet Program. For example, given that this 1,000-calorie-a-day menu would inspire impressive weight loss in any woman, if you are a man or do not need to lose much weight, feel free to add a few extra servings of whatever whole foods you desire. If you are a cancer or heart patient or someone with risk factors for developing heart disease, it would be to your advantage to make fish your only animal fat.

If you do want to eat foods from other animal sources, *be sure they are grass fed*, because corn-fed animals have a much higher omega-6 to omega-3 fatty acid ratio, which has repeatedly been shown to increase your risk for developing heart disease and cancer. The animals should preferably be organically raised, so that you are not consuming cloned animals or those fed genetically engineered corn. Although this may at first seem radical or extremely prudent to the average person who was raised on processed fast foods, it is how most people in the rest of the world eat. The Rice Diet is what the majority of people in developing nations consume, because whatever grows out of the ground is the only food available to them. They do not have access to convenience foods that are highly processed and loaded with plasticized fats (a food scientist's name for hydrogenated fats!), sodium-rich additives, and man-made mutations and chemicals galore. Don't forget that whole, unprocessed foods are what most centenarians eat. So let's get back to the basics with the weekly menus that follow.

Weekly Menus

Meal Week 1 Summer	Sunday 1,000 Calories (±100 Calories)	Monday 800 Calories (±100 Calories)	Tuesday 1,000 Calories (±100 Calories)
Breakfast	1 Banana Breakfast Muffin* 1 cup soy or nonfat milk 1 medium orange	1 cup oatmeal 2 tablespoons raisins 1 cup berries 1 cup green tea	2 cups Puffed Kashi 1 tablespoon freshly ground flaxseed 1 cup soy or nonfat milk ½ medium banana
Lunch	⅔ cup Barley Mushroom Soup* 1 slice Ezekiel 4:9 toast 2 cups mixed baby greens, shredded carrots, cherry tomatoes, and broccoli sprouts 1 tablespoon chopped walnuts Balsamic vinegar and herbs	2 Banana Breakfast Muffins* ½ cup frozen grapes	⅔ cup Barley Mushroom Soup* 2 cups mesclun or spring mix salad, cherry tomatoes, and broccoli sprouts Balsamic vinegar 1 teaspoon olive oil and herbs 1 peach
Dinner	1 Black Bean Burger with Fresh Salsa* 1 cup Napa Slaw with Honey Mustard* 2 Medjool dates	⅔ cup jasmine rice 1 cup watermelon 1 cup blueberries	1 cup Roasted Red Pepper Bisque* 1 cup jasmine rice ½ cup mango chunks 1 cup blueberries

An asterisk indicates that the recipe is included in this book.

Wednesday 1,000 Calories (±100 Calories)	Thursday 1,000 Calories (±100 Calories)	Friday 1,000 Calories (±100 Calories)	Saturday 1,000 Calories (±100 Calories)
⅓ cup granola 6 ounces plain low-fat or nonfat yogurt 1 tablespoon freshly ground flaxseed 1 cup orange segments	1 cup flaked cereal 1 cup soy or nonfat milk 1 tablespoon freshly ground flaxseed 1 cup berries	1 cup shredded wheat 1 cup soy or nonfat milk 1 tablespoon raisins 1 peach	3 3-inch Banana Berry Oatmeal Pancakes* ¼ cup Berry Puree*
1 Black Bean Burger with Fresh Salsa* 1 cup Napa Slaw with Honey Mustard* 2 Medjool dates	¾ cup Hummus in a Hurry* 2 cups raw veggie strips 1 cup pineapple chunks	2 cups roasted vegetables 1 whole-wheat tortilla 2 cups assorted green salad and choice of toppings 1 tablespoon pumpkin seeds 1 teaspoon olive oil Balsamic vinegar	1 cup pasta with ½ cup no-salt spaghetti sauce 1 cup baby spinach salad with ½ cup mandarin orange segments 1 tablespoon walnuts Balsamic vinegar and herbs
½ cup Hummus in a Hurry* 3 cups raw veggie strips 1 cup frozen grapes	1 cup Roasted Red Pepper Bisque* 1 cup brown rice 1 cup roasted vegetables 1 cup watermelon	1 cup pasta with ½ cup no-salt spaghetti sauce Garden salad 1 teaspoon olive oil Balsamic vinegar	3 ounces grilled tempeh on ½ cup quinoa, topped with 2 tablespoons no-salt barbecue sauce 1½ cups grilled vegetables 1 cup mango chunks and blueberries

(continued)

Weekly Menus (*continued*)

Meal Week 2 Fall	Sunday 1,000 Calories (±100 Calories)	Monday 800 Calories (±100 Calories)	Tuesday 1,000 Calories (±100 Calories)

Breakfast	2 cups Puffed Kashi
	1 cup soy or
	  nonfat milk
	1 tablespoon freshly
	  ground flaxseed
	1 tablespoon dried
	  cherries
	½ small banana
		2 slices Banana
		  Barley Bread*
		1 cup fresh fruit
		1 cup green tea
			1 cup flaked cereal
			1 cup soy or nonfat
			  milk
			½ cup mixed berries
			1 tablespoon dried
			  cherries

Lunch	1¼ cups Kasha
	  Varnishkes*
	2 cups romaine
	  lettuce
	1 orange
	1 teaspoon olive oil
	Balsamic vinegar
		⅔ cup brown rice
		2 cups fruit salad
			1¼ cups Kasha
			  Varnishkes*
			2 slices Nancy's
			  Baked Eggplant*
			1 pear

Dinner	2 slices Nancy's
	  Baked Eggplant*
	⅓ cup brown rice
	1 cup steamed
	  broccoflower
	1 cup seasonal fruit
	  salad
		Fruit smoothie (2
		  cups fruit)
		⅔ cup brown rice
			1 cup polenta
			½ cup no-salt
			  spaghetti sauce
			1 cup steamed
			  broccoflower
			1 cup seasonal
			  fruit salad

Wednesday 1,000 Calories (±100 Calories)	Thursday 1,000 Calories (±100 Calories)	Friday 1,000 Calories (±100 Calories)	Saturday 1,000 Calories (±100 Calories)
2 slices Banana Barley Bread* ½ cup orange mango juice	1 cup Cream of Wheat 1 tablespoon raisins 1 tablespoon freshly ground flaxseed ½ cup orange mango juice	1 cup oatmeal 1 tablespoon raisins 1 tablespoon freshly ground flaxseed 1 cup berries	2 3-inch Banana Berry Oatmeal Pancakes* ¼ cup Berry Puree*
1 cup polenta ½ cup no-salt spaghetti sauce Big tossed salad Balsamic vinegar and herbs 1 cup seasonal fruit salad	1 cup Cassandra's Carrot Ginger Soup* ⅔ cup brown rice ½ cup brussels sprouts 1 pear	2 cups Barley and Black-Eyed Pea Salad* 1 cup brussels sprouts 1 apple	½ can Health Valley Vegetarian Chili (add 1 tablespoon fresh lime juice and freshly chopped cilantro and jalapeño as desired) 6 organic no-salt corn chips 2 cups tossed salad Apple slices Balsamic vinegar and herbs Fresh fruit smoothie (1 cup ice and 1 cup fruit)
1 cup Cassandra's Carrot Ginger Soup* ⅔ cup brown rice ½ cup brussels sprouts ¾ cup nonfat yogurt Apple slices	1½ cups Barley and Black-Eyed Pea Salad* 1 cup spinach salad 1 cup frozen mango chunks 1 cup nonfat yogurt	1 cup cooked pasta with ¼ cup sun-dried tomato marinara Big tossed salad 1 teaspoon olive oil Balsamic vinegar 1 baked pear	1½ cups Dr. Rosati's Pasta con Sarde* 2 cups spinach salad ½ cup mandarin orange segments Balsamic vinegar

(continued)

Weekly Menus (continued)

Meal Week 3 Winter	Sunday 1,000 Calories (±100 Calories)	Monday 800 Calories (±100 Calories)	Tuesday 1,000 Calories (±100 Calories)
Breakfast	2 Nancy's Carrot Muffins* 6 ounces nonfat yogurt 1 tablespoon freshly ground flaxseed 1 cup frozen mango chunks	1 cup oatmeal 1 tablespoon raisins 1 cup mixed berries 1 cup green tea	1 cup shredded wheat 1 cup soy or nonfat milk 1 tablespoon raisins 1 medium banana
Lunch	½ Spaghetti Squash with Honey Mustard Sauce* ½ cup Bayou Bourbon Baked Beans* 1 cup Braised Bok Choy*	1 cup brown rice 1 apple 1 medium banana	1 Sweet Potato Burger* with sliced onion, balsamic vinegar, and no-salt ketchup 1 cup Braised Bok Choy*
Dinner	1 Sweet Potato Burger* with sliced onion, balsamic vinegar, and no-salt ketchup Sliced tomato 1 teaspoon olive oil 1 cup frozen mixed berries	1 cup Citrus-Kissed Quinoa* ½ cup frozen mango chunks	1½ cups Turkish Lentil-Tomato Soup* 1 cup Jicama, Radish, and Cucumber Salad* 2 Medjool dates 1 tablespoon walnuts

Wednesday 1,000 Calories (±100 Calories)	Thursday 1,000 Calories (±100 Calories)	Friday 1,000 Calories (±100 Calories)	Saturday 1,000 Calories (±100 Calories)
⅓ cup granola 6 ounces plain nonfat yogurt 1 teaspoon freshly ground flaxseed 1 cup grapes	2 cups Puffed Kashi 1 cup soy or nonfat milk 1 tablespoon freshly ground flaxseed 1 tablespoon dried apricots 1 small banana	⅓ cup granola 6 ounces plain yogurt 1 cup frozen grapes	1 Nancy's Carrot Muffin* Fresh fruit smoothie (1 cup nonfat yogurt and 1 cup fruit)
1 cup Turkish Lentil-Tomato Soup* 1 matzo cracker 1 cup Jicama, Radish, and Cucumber Salad* 1 apple	Leftover Chinese restaurant food: 1 cup steamed rice 1½ cups stir-fried vegetables and tofu with extra ginger, garlic, lemon, and sake; no salt	1½ cups Spicy Thai Stir-Fry* over ⅔ cup whole-wheat noodles 1 cup Nancy's Ambrosia*	1 cup Bayou Baked Bourbon Beans* 1 cup Napa Slaw with Honey Mustard* 1 cup berries
Chinese food, eaten out: 1 cup steamed rice 1½ cups stir-fried vegetables and tofu Order with extra ginger, garlic, lemon, and sake; no salt	1½ cups Spicy Thai Stir-Fry* 1½ cups whole-wheat noodles 1 cup Nancy's Ambrosia*	3 ounces Rice House Fried Fish* 1 baked potato, small 1 cup Napa Slaw with Honey Mustard*	3 ounces Rice House Fried Fish* ½ cup Citrus-Kissed Quinoa* 1 cup steamed green beans with fresh chopped basil 1 poached pear in pomegranate juice

(continued)

Weekly Menus (*continued*)

Meal **Week 4** Spring	Sunday 1,000 Calories (±100 Calories)	Monday 800 Calories (±100 Calories)	Tuesday 1,000 Calories (±100 Calories)
Breakfast	1 cup Kashi cereal 1 cup nonfat, plain Greek yogurt 1 cup blueberries 1 tablespoon freshly ground flaxseed	1 cup oatmeal 3 prunes 1 peach, frozen, sliced 1 cup green tea	1 cup shredded wheat 1 cup soy or nonfat milk 1 tablespoon freshly ground flaxseed 1 cup mixed berries
Lunch	3 ounces shrimp, sautéed with honey and lemon 1½ cups stir-fried vegetables 1½ cups rice noodles 1 teaspoon Worcestershire sauce ½ teaspoon toasted sesame oil	⅔ cup brown rice with tomato basil dressing 1 sliced apple 1 cup pineapple chunks	1 whole-wheat pita bread ½ cup tuna (canned, no salt, in spring water) 2 tablespoons nonfat yogurt Chopped tomato Fresh chopped dill Cracked black pepper 1 cup grapes
Dinner	1 cup White Beans and Greens* 1 cup pasta 1 poached pear in pomegranate juice	1¼ cups Berry-Barley Fruited Salad*	1 Stuffed Cooked Tomato* 1 cup cooked kale with vegetable stock and cracked black pepper

Wednesday 1,000 Calories (±100 Calories)	Thursday 1,000 Calories (±100 Calories)	Friday 1,000 Calories (±100 Calories)	Saturday 1,000 Calories (±100 Calories)
1 cup hot oat-bran cereal 1 cup soy or nonfat milk 1 tablespoon freshly ground flaxseed 2 tablespoons raisins ¼ teaspoon cinnamon	1 cup steel-cut oats 1 small banana 1 tablespoon dried cherries 1 tablespoon freshly ground flaxseed 1 cup soy or non-fat milk	⅓ cup granola ½ cup Puffed Kamut 1 cup nonfat, plain Greek yogurt 1 tablespoon freshly ground flaxseed 1 peach, frozen, sliced	Omelet: 1 egg, 2 egg whites with sautéed green and red peppers and onions 1 cup roasted red potato wedges with fresh chopped rosemary 1 cup honeydew melon
1 Stuffed Cooked Tomato* 1 cup cooked kale with vegetable stock and cracked black pepper 1 poached pear in pomegranate juice	1 serving Refried Beans and Salsa with 6 Chips* 2 cups raw veggies 1 cup strawberries	1 baked potato 3 cups raw veggies (salad bar choices, without salt) Balsamic or other vinegar 1 pear	Salad: 2 cups arugula ½ cup roasted beets 1 tablespoon walnuts 1 sliced pear ⅓ cup garbanzo beans 1 slice Ezekiel 4:9 bread with 1 teaspoon olive oil and 2 tablespoons nutritional yeast
1 serving Refried Beans and Salsa with 6 Chips* 1 cup raw veggies 1 peach	1 cup White Beans and Greens* 1 cup Berry-Barley Fruited Salad*	3 ounces grilled salmon topped with 1 table-spoon honey and chili powder 1 cup Mashed Cauliflower* 1 cup grilled red potatoes and vegetables 1 cup strawberries	1½ cups Rice House Mushroom Stuffing* Tossed salad 1 teaspoon olive oil Balsamic vinegar 1 cup fresh fruit salad

You will also notice that each week's menu is reflective of a season of the year. This is done to illustrate and sensitize you to the availability of certain fruits and vegetables at different times of the year. Since you will likely be using these menus for four consecutive weeks, the suggested fruits and vegetables may not be what are freshest and most affordable, so be ready to make locally grown substitutions. For instance, in January, we find that the available tomatoes and bell peppers are basically inedible and expensive, so we substitute with sundried tomatoes and enjoy stuffed acorn or butternut squash instead of stuffed peppers. Think fresh, local, and organic when making any substitutions.

A daily multivitamin/mineral supplement is recommended, as well as 500 to 1,000 mg of calcium (depending on your calcium-rich food consumption), especially if you have osteopenia (a reduction in bone density), osteoporosis, or a history of osteoporosis in your family.

Rice Diet Tips for Certain Conditions

Overweight: Eat a lot (four to six half-cup servings) of organic vegetables. Eat whole, unprocessed foods without added salt, sugar, and hydrogenated fats; limit animal fats. Enjoy a variety of organic and preferably locally grown whole grains, beans, and fruits, as well as a serving of low-fat dairy products, or seafood daily.

Hypertensive: Follow the same tips as for the overweight category, with an added focus on, and commitment to, avoiding added sodium in foods and increasing your intake of potassium-rich fresh fruits, vegetables, and legumes. Fresh fruits and vegetables contain more potassium than frozen and significantly more than canned ones, so, again, fresh is usually best. Because no-salt substitutes that contain potassium chloride will continue to train your taste buds

(continued)

and your mind to think that foods should taste salty to be good, they are not recommended. Healthier and more flavorful seasonings are fresh herbs, spices, lemon, lime, and vinegars. If you still want to use no-salt substitutes that contain potassium chloride, ask your physician whether it would be contraindicated for you, as too high of a potassium level can be dangerous.

Hypercholesterolemic and diabetic: Follow the same tips as for the overweight category, with an added focus on increasing the amount of soluble fiber–rich oats, beans or peas, and barley. Two to three servings of these foods per day will produce therapeutic improvements in your cholesterol and your blood-sugar levels and stability. Garlic, onions, olive oil, and fish have been shown to improve people's lipid panels (fat tests that include cholesterol, HDLs, and triglycerides), and these foods, plus cinnamon, would benefit anyone who is concerned about diabetes.

Heart disease, cancer, and arthritis sufferers and healthy people seeking to prevent chronic diseases: Assume the same smart preventive strategies outlined in the overweight category and further reduce your disease risks and inflammation processes and enhance your immune system by increasing your intake of broccoli sprouts (the highest source of the chemical precursor to sulforaphane, a cancer fighter), vitamin C–rich citrus fruits and tomatoes, and vitamin A–rich foods that are usually dark orange, red, or green in color; omega-3 fatty acid–rich flaxseeds, walnuts, soybeans, and fish are also health-promoting staples, especially salmon and the smaller, oilier fish, such as sardines, herring, and unsalted anchovies.

Whether you have health problems or just want to responsibly do everything you can to prevent them, commit to this

(continued)

dietary challenge for a month and experience how the food you choose can change the way you feel for the better. If you are on medications or have medical concerns, see your doctor before beginning this healthy diet and request blood work if you have not done so recently. Comparing your blood work before beginning the Rice Diet and one month into it will inspire you beyond your wildest expectations. There is nothing like dramatic physical results to encourage people to embrace long-term lifestyle changes.

Your Food Pledge

One way to become conscious of, and responsible for, how and what you eat is by making a food pledge. This can be as simple as the following:

> I will eat a wholesome diet with very low sodium, sugar, and saturated fat for one month to see what power I have in creating the results I want for _____.

This can be made more specific:

> I will eat whole foods, which include all grains, beans, fruits, and vegetables, with a daily seafood or organic nonfat dairy (soy or rice milk) choice for one month to experience the power I have to influence _____.

Eating the Mindful Way

Although the menus in this chapter are designed to give you a sense of food and portion sizes that would provide a 1,000-calorie diet, if you wish to consume 100 to 200 calories more, you will still lose weight, but it will be at a slower pace unless you exercise more. Many people like the idea of having set portion sizes, but soon realize that by keeping a food log and gaining more experience with listening to their bodies, they have become mindful of what, when, and why they are eating and less fixated on portion size.

Other basic strategies for success include not skipping meals, especially breakfast. If my schedule changes and challenges my ability to eat when I need to, I always have some fruit, a box of shredded wheat cereal, or something healthy available nearby, to avoid the inevitable pitfalls that could await me. Always consider vegetables the preferred food group to seek second and third servings from. Vegetables contain many fewer calories than any other food group does, plus they contain a lot of vitamins, minerals, and fiber. One habit that has helped me maintain my desired weight, after childbirth and menopause, is to start my dinners (and often lunches) with a couple of cups of tossed salad. Eating this much fiber and bulk first greatly reduces how much I will eat of higher-calorie foods that follow the salad.

As you can see from the sample menus, whole, clean foods can provide a wide and interesting variety of choices. Although many of us prefer a diverse selection of foods during the week, others are happier and often more successful with simple, repetitive choices. While the majority of the dishes are simply prepared, they do incorporate leftovers for lunch and some examples of healthier restaurant foods to enjoy for a change of pace.

In choosing a restaurant, it's best to consider those that prepare foods "in house"; if the restaurant prepares its dishes from scratch, the chef can easily cook meals with no added salt. This is the case with most good, authentic Italian restaurants. To enhance your success there, it's often best to simply ask the waiter which fresh vegetables and fish are available, rather than choosing from the menu. Ask that your food be grilled with a teaspoon of olive oil, some fresh lemon juice, and herbs; request that no salt or sauces be added. Other tips for restaurant success include asking for one slice of bread, rather than an entire basket, and, instead of using butter, requesting olive oil. Being clear on what you truly want before you enter the restaurant is key; this can save you from making choices you may later regret. In fact, if you call the restaurant beforehand to make sure that it can prepare a vegetarian or seafood dish without salt, this is really exercising your power, which is crucial to co-creating the good health and the weight you desire.

Regardless of what situation you find yourself in, always remember that if your priority is to eat something low in sodium and saturated fat that you will enjoy, you need to ask for it in a way that can be heard. Once I attended a round-table luncheon at a national cardiac conference. When I walked into the room and saw that they were serving beef stroganoff, I quickly engaged a server and admitted that I was a vegetarian who had unfortunately forgotten to request a special meal in advance, as I was accustomed to doing at such events. I immediately apologized for any inconvenience that I was creating for him and asked whether he had any fresh fish or vegetables that I might have instead. He came back, grinning from ear to ear, with the most beautiful salmon, served with steamed broccoli, a baked potato, and a salad! Of course, I tipped him generously, and we both had a win-win experience. The cardiologists at the table looked at their less-than-healthy lunch and then at my tasty, nutritious meal and asked, "How did you get that?" I replied honestly, "I asked for it." That's what can happen when you take responsibility for co-creating what you want and acting on that desire!

Although eating in restaurants, at conferences, and on the road can be challenging, you can enhance your odds of eating health-promoting foods that you will enjoy if you plan ahead and shop and pack wisely. Research shows that people who planned their menus and shopped accordingly consumed far more healthy fruits and vegetables than did individuals who did not plan ahead. Stocking your pantry, car, and office with no-salt-added staples and snacks can be incredibly helpful; surrounding yourself with optimal food items makes choosing them ever so much easier. The often-quoted excuses "Well, there was nothing else I could eat" or "I didn't have any healthier choices there" are really rather lame. We always have the choice to eat or take a healthy option with us, rather than to unconsciously set ourselves up to not have one.

One impetus to improve the quality of our diet and transform our relationship with food is hearing from others who have taken these steps and are now reaping the rewards we desire. One Ricer recently returned with photos of his pantry, documenting his "before" and "after" Rice Diet conversion experience. The photos of his former pantry showed that his cupboards were chock-full of processed foods; the after photos revealed a cupboard filled with a variety of staples that facilitated his continued success. He made a choice, and he acted on it.

Other Ricers have said that while at the program, they met cooks who specialized in healthy cuisine; when they discovered that these cooks lived near them, they later hired them to deliver Rice Diet foods to their home. This inspired others to advertise at their local health food stores for cooks to provide meals from Rice Diet recipes. Although hiring a cook to make your meals may sound extravagant, these Ricers actually discovered that they saved money because they were not eating in restaurants as often, and they no longer needed to pay for doctor visits or costly prescriptions. There are other ways to ensure that your meals are healthy without spending too much time planning or cooking. For many years, while I was single and primarily cooked for one to two people, I enjoyed very inexpensive and healthy meals by always having a large fresh salad and a bean and vegetable dish ready. Regardless of your family's size, it's helpful to cook enough for three to four meals and also to have ready-made, convenient leftovers handy—such as baked potatoes and sweet potatoes, roasted winter squashes, and a variety of vegetables.

Some Ricers, inspired by our organic farm tours, have returned home and joined community-supported agriculture farms that deliver organic foods that were picked fresh that morning. They describe these food deliveries as the highlight of their week. Others have enthusiastically related how they organized healthy dinner clubs, as well as slow food fund-raiser dinners on local farms, which became wholly engaging eating experiences. As you become more familiar with the foods that you will be eating and the rhythm of your new *dieta*, it will become second nature for you to prepare your meals, find others to cook with, and discover other cost-effective ways to have your healthy meals prepared.

Your *Dieta* Journal

Your *Dieta* Journal is an invaluable tool to help you become mindful of what you eat and to record your progress in actualizing your intentions. It will allow you to understand and keep track of your food intake and daily exercise regime and will introduce you to a new and effective way of noticing your thoughts and feelings. Through journalizing, you can assess and visualize where you are and where you want to be with your food and lifestyle choices. For anyone who is diabetic or familiar with that food exchange system or the one outlined in my previous books, you may want to convert your portions into these familiar serving sizes. Otherwise, simply documenting your food and guesstimating serving sizes will greatly enhance your ability to consume consciously. Commit to doing so every day for one month.

For those of you who do not want to concern yourselves with the fact that a teaspoon of oil averages 5 grams of fat (and thus 45 calories) and is often found naturally within every ounce of animal product and cereal and to a lesser degree in most servings of vegetables and fruits—you don't have to. It is certainly easier to be healthy and lean if you choose simple, whole foods and limit your high-fat foods to 1–2 teaspoons of oil per day or a couple of table-spoons of nuts or seeds per day. Remember that eating processed foods with hidden fats, sodium, and sugar is a recipe for obesity and chronic disease!

Take a look at the sample *Dieta* Journal on the next page. The tallies stand for the following: S, starch; V, vegetables; Fr, fruit; P, protein; D, dairy; and F, fat.

Your Diet Plan: 1,000 Calories

Date: 5/9/09

Today's Weight: 243 pounds   **Blood Pressure/Other: 160/98**

	Food	Cal	Fat (g)	Sodium (mg)
Breakfast	½ cup oatmeal	80	1	0
	1 cup skim milk	90	0	120
	½ banana	60	1	1
	Total	230	3	121

S = __1__   V = _____   Fr = __1__   P = _____   D = __1__   F = _____

	Food	Cal	Fat (g)	Sodium (mg)
Lunch	1 cup brown rice	232	2	0
	1 teaspoon olive oil	45	5	
	1 cup steamed broccoli	46	1	41
	1⅓ cups strawberries	66	1	3
	Total	389	9	44

S = __3__   V = __2__   Fr = __1__   P = _____   D = _____   F = _____

	Food	Cal	Fat (g)	Sodium (mg)
Dinner	3 ounces cooked snapper	109	2	48
	½ cup potato	80	0	5
	2 cups tossed salad	40	0	71
	½ cup stewed tomatoes	35	0	31
	1 cup fruit sorbet	240	0	22
	Total	504	2	177

S = __1__   V = __3__   Fr = __3__   P = __3__   D = _____   F = __1__

	Cal	Fat (g)	Sodium (mg)
Daily Total for Calories / Fat (g) / Sodium (mg):	1,123	13	342

Total Daily Servings

Starch = __5__   Vegetables = __5__   Fruit = __4__

Protein = __3__   Dairy = __1__   Fat = __1__

(continued)

Your Diet Plan: 1,000 Calories (*continued*)

Meal Plan Goals	Actual Intake	Differences (+/−) between Goals and Intake
S = 5	5	____
V = 5	5	____
Fr = 3	6	+3　(from fruit sorbet's 240 calories, which contains 180 calories more than a 60-calorie fruit)
P = 3	3	____
D = 1	1	____
F = 1	1	____

Daily Activity	Goal	Actual
Cardiovascular	60 minutes daily	60 minutes
Strength training	30 minutes twice weekly	20 minutes
Flexibility (stretching)	5–10 minutes daily	10 minutes
Mind/body relaxation	30 minutes daily	60 minutes

Personal Notes

Today I attended the journalizing class at the Rice Diet Program. I frankly wasn't expecting much from the experience but was amazed at what came up for me. When I asked myself where the last fifty pounds had come from . . . I didn't know that I had the answer until I started writing about the safety my excess weight was providing me, increasingly, since my assault. I was shocked that there was any connection between the two! My New Year's resolution is to journalize daily!! P.S. That fruit sorbet was no-fat, but those 240 calories were sure not as nutritious, satisfying, or filling as 4 cups of cold watermelon would have been.

For more nutritional details, go to www.ricediet.com and download some complimentary sections of our *Journal for Health: A Workbook for the Rice Diet*, which includes blank journal pages, an extensive reference for food exchanges, and charts for tracking your health parameters and improvements. If you prefer to use the original workbook, filled with other supportive journalizing information, you can order one from www.ricedietstore.com.

Exercise: Do What You *Will* Do

Enjoying daily exercise is a close second to "clean eating" for producing positive physical results fast. So a key component to your Rice *Dieta* will be integrating daily exercise into your life. When Ricers ask me, "What is the best exercise to do?" my answer is always the same: "Whatever you *will* do!"

Enjoying what you do is always the best advice I know. We generally encourage participants to increase their activity slowly and gradually, building up to one hour per day of aerobic exercise to get themselves going. Once your body adapts to this daily physical activity, you may want to increase the duration of time and give yourself a wider variety of activities.

For many people, especially those who are not at all accustomed to exercising, walking is the best way to begin. (Water walking may suit you better if you've recently had physical challenges or any orthopedic concerns.) Walking is free, available anywhere, beneficial to your cardiovascular system, effective at expending calories and reducing stress, and enjoyable for those who choose for it to be. I say the latter because few people seem to be exempt from inertia; most of us have to make a conscious choice to get out the door despite our borderline depression, rainy weather, or whatever condition we allow to impede our commitment to exercise.

Unless exercise becomes a habit, as deeply engrained as brushing your teeth, our resolve can crumble at the most insignificant excuse. When I have a big project with a deadline in the near future, I am even more committed to walk an hour at least six days per week. Otherwise, I am more vulnerable to feeling the symptoms of unreleased stress: back spasms, joint stiffness, and mental fogginess or fatigue. If people need to speak with me, I have a common response: "I'll be glad to talk with you if you want to walk with me at 8:10 a.m., right after I take my son to school."

If someone is trying to book an appointment with me for that hallowed time of day, I habitually say, "I'd like to see you, but I already have something scheduled between 8 and 9:30." This is the truth; I don't have to elaborate that it's a daily appointment to walk with myself.

You may choose to do the same. Walking forty-five to sixty minutes each day is time you spend taking care of yourself. It not only boosts any weight loss you are trying to accomplish, but it also improves your mind-body balance, your sense of well-being, and your clarity of thought.

Beyond Walking

Walking never goes out of style, but as you become more fit, you may want a more intense cardio challenge. For those of you who are near your goal weight and are without orthopedic problems, you may enjoy a jog or a run. If you are in this club, remember to gradually replace your walking time with a walk/run, starting with five minutes today and ten minutes tomorrow. Listen to your body; many of us have discovered that walking will get us to the same place that running will, with less chance of injury.

Swimming, biking, and inline skating are all wonderful cardio workouts. For those of you who play sports, such as tennis or cross-country skiing (in the winter, of course), you can break up your walking routine—and wake up your muscles and circulatory system—by alternating your cardio workout. My Pilates instructor recently reintroduced me to the hula hoop. I couldn't believe that I instantly remembered how to do it, after a forty-five-year sabbatical. And what a workout! For a couple of dollars, you could buy a water-filled hula hoop—a large one for your waist area and a smaller one for your arms will provide a great full-body workout and you won't need a gym membership or waste time and gas driving yourself elsewhere. It's invaluable to have these lying around to reduce your excuses about why you can't work out. You always can.

A few new dance-inspired classes are becoming all the rage in certain communities around the country. Zumba and Nia are fun, dancelike classes that incorporate stretching (see how important stretching is on the next page) and cardio, both to the beat of music! Our closest gym is now offering Zumba, which features aerobic fitness routines, with a combination of fast and slow rhythms that tone and sculpt the body. Moving to a fusion of Latin and international music makes a workout more fun than you can believe!

As you heal your body, you will also heal any previous thoughts and beliefs that exercise can't be fun.

Cross-Training for Better Health

On the second page of your *Dieta* Journal, record your daily exercise. As noted, I've recommended that once you're ready to move beyond walking or add more dimensions to your workout, you can increase the benefits of weight loss and health goals by cross-training, which means adding strength training, stretching, and flexibility exercises, as well as mind-body relaxation.

> *Strengthening*: As you get older, it becomes absolutely essential to keep your body strong. A natural effect of aging is the loss of muscle and bone mass, so on your new road to health (and, dare I say, longevity) you need to pay extra attention to both. Lifting free weights and working out with Therabands (plastic stretchy strips) at home are great ways to tone without much cost or time spent commuting to a gym. And mixing this up with Pilates, yoga, and a "body pump" class (a blend of cardio and weight lifting that is fast and fun and makes your body pump with energy!) can give you a variety of ways to enjoy yourself—while strengthening your bones and muscles.

> *Flexibility and stretching*: In order for your muscles and joints to stay healthy and mobile, it's important to stretch these areas of your body. Yoga and Pilates incorporate all-over body and joint stretches through their movements and asanas (yoga poses). But there are many ways to stretch. Yoga balls and firm rollers are a great home remedy for your flexibility and stretching needs; they are also invaluable in sustaining a healthy back without weekly massage therapy sessions, which are wonderful but costly.

Mind-body balance and relaxation: The more scientists delve into the positive, life-enhancing effects of exercise, the more evidence is discovered about how your mind also benefits from physical activity. The upshot? You need to rest, relax, and recuperate, but you also need to strengthen your mind-body balance. In addition to yoga, another ancient Eastern form of exercise offers an immediate and fruitful way of uniting body and mind—tai chi. Tai chi chuan is a very rich and profound system of mental, emotional, spiritual, and physical development. Its roots stretch back more than three thousand years, and it is based on many aspects of Chinese culture: medicine, martial arts, cultivation of personal energy, Taoist philosophy, meditation, and calisthenics. Although most people associate tai chi with groups of people exercising with slow, synchronized movements in public parks, other aspects of the art are seated and standing meditation and a wide range of auxiliary exercises that include stretching, joint warm-ups, massage, breathing, "core" (torso) work, and movements based on the imitation of animals.

How You Will Feel

If you have followed the diet now for even a day or two, you will undoubtedly have noticed some results. While men each lose an average of thirty pounds and women an average of nineteen pounds in the first four weeks, during the next few months, a weight loss of one to three and a half pounds per week is very doable, depending on your weight to begin with. Don't be alarmed if you need to visit the bathroom often; a no-salt-added diet will cause you to urinate the excess water from your body if you have been consuming too much sodium. Your body is exquisitely designed to take in or excrete the amount of fluids necessary to maintain health, depending on the sodium you have ingested.

Along with this initial rapid weight loss, you may soon notice that your joints feel more fluid or less stiff, you may be sleeping more soundly, your headaches may have disappeared (especially if you have reduced or eliminated your coffee-, tea-, or soda-drinking habits), and your energy level may have changed. Note any of these physical changes on the bottom of the second page of your *Dieta* Journal. Although some people are surprised at the burst of energy they feel on the diet, for many others this response is obvious only after a week of their feeling less energetic, due to detoxing any number of deleterious substances that they have previously habitually consumed. For instance, people who stop a caffeine habit cold turkey will often have headaches for a few days, but "this, too, will pass" after the first week of detox. (Of course, participants are offered the options of going cold turkey, titrating themselves off caffeine, or taking a headache medication.) Keep your eyes on the prize. And if you are tired, take a nap or go to bed earlier. Listen to your body for a change of pace . . . it is ready to talk to you!

Cleansing your body builds the physical platform for you to begin healing at the core, and it will support the exploration of your emotional, mental, and spiritual growth in the upcoming three chapters.

Now that your body has so quickly shown you its ability and willingness to heal and to make you feel better, the next chapter, "Healing Your Heart," will enroll the body part that can effectively enhance the duration of your great passions. Although in the past you likely made most of your food choices unconsciously, you can become newly aware of your attitudes toward food and eating and let go of any negativity that may inhibit your efforts to lose weight and get healthy. The following chapter will introduce you to ways to uncover and release any emotional blocks that could prevent you from truly embracing your ability to take care of yourself, cherish yourself, and treat all of your being as a vessel of love. You will begin to understand why Ricers often start their "shares" with "This is not a diet but a *dieta*, a way of life that has transformed me."

Congratulations on taking your first step into the physical realm, and welcome to the upcoming exploration that will empower your heart!

3

Healing Your Heart

*Love many things, for therein lies the true strength, and
whosoever loves much performs much, and can accomplish
much, and what is done in love is done well.*
—Vincent Van Gogh

This chapter enables you to focus on your feelings so that you
can maximize the emotional experiences that empower you and
heal the feelings that get in your way and prevent you from attaining true health. We know that feelings can create disease just as
dramatically as an unhealthy diet can, although often much less
obviously. A big part of gaining control of your emotions—or the
power that you've unconsciously allowed them to have over you—is
your ability to become aware of, and then responsible for, your
feelings.

The first tool you encounter in these pages will help you understand your relationship with food. How do you think about food?

What was your family's attitude toward food? Was food used as an expression of love or as punishment? Did your mother restrict food or force you to eat it even if you didn't like it? Did she obsess about calories or your body weight? How might this attitude have affected you? These are some of the questions you will begin to examine so that you can redefine your relationship with food and discover a joy in eating that is fruitful and supportive.

In this chapter you will explore your feelings, how you can become aware of them, and which senses help you best shift them; then you will consciously choose to perceive and feel things differently, in a way that empowers you, rather than defeats you.

When you journalize your results, this will reveal which sensory approaches and practices facilitate your positive emotional shifts most effectively. As research has now repeatedly shown, positive states of mind trigger an upward spiral within us that leads to growth and epitomizes flourishing. Who wouldn't want an extra serving of flourishing, thriving, and prospering? Yes, we are talking about optimizing your life potential, not only by improving your physical health but also by taking the tremendous power that comes from recognizing and controlling your feelings in order to inspire and expand your mind and your world.

Explore Your Emotional Relationship with Food

During my first six weeks of working at the Rice Diet Program, I learned more about my relationship with food than I had previously understood in two decades of being a semivegetarian "health nut." Although most people would have labeled me a conscious consumer, and I admit that I would have proudly done so myself, it was not until my fifth week of following the Rice Diet that I experienced a huge epiphany about emotional eating. I was still doing some nutrition consulting at the time, and I was going to a great deal of trouble to carry my food with me to various locations in three counties as I traveled to meet with clients. Despite the extra effort, I was determined to eat only food allowed on the Rice Diet for at least six weeks to see what the average Ricer was experiencing. If I expected participants to follow this discipline, I felt that I should do so as well, to fully appreciate what the diet was like in every way possible. So when I found myself at my favorite bakery, three-fourths of the way through a big, chunky brownie, I stopped short. It suddenly dawned on me that the reason for my being in the bakery—without a conscious thought or plan—was that moments earlier, someone had hurt my feelings. This was the first time in my life that I realized that I was totally unconscious of what I was eating, and that I was eating in response to an emotional upset; I had turned to my drug of choice—chocolate—to assuage my hurt.

Despite more than a decade of attending nutrition conferences where we examined unconscious, emotionally inspired eating, I never thought they were talking about me! I thought this behavior applied to overweight people, not to everyone to various degrees. This experience helped me better understand and appreciate that regardless of our weight, we *all* eat for emotional reasons at times. Some people may do this more often and regularly than others do, but it's the same behavior. And at the root of this behavior is the fact that our emotions can hijack our brains, prompting us to consume foods without awareness. The good news is that we can become mindful and choose to attend to the root of the problem, rather than perpetuate a habit of numbing out with food.

Most of us are aware of a food or numerous foods that we turn to for solace, for comfort, or as an anesthetic. You may already be aware of which comfort foods you prefer for distraction, for celebration, or to alleviate sadness. Becoming a conscious eater and aligning your physical responses with your expanding mental and emotional awareness are all essential steps for choosing a healthy *dieta*.

One day in a Rice Diet Program group, a man showed up for a meeting that my husband, Dr. Bob Rosati, was conducting, and said, "I don't know what you're talking about in here today, but I don't believe in all that psychological stuff!"

Bob said, "We're just getting to know one another, sharing a bit about our families and how we were raised."

The man responded by summarizing how he had a loving mother, father, brother, and sister. He elaborated on how everyone was pretty busy, ate on different schedules, but always came together at one o'clock on Sunday afternoons in a Chinese restaurant down the street from their house. When he shared the latter half of this last sentence, his voice cracked and his eyes teared up. He was unable to mask the emotions he didn't even know he had about how precious and few the hours were with his entire family together.

He then gradually admitted that even while he was on the program here, every Sunday afternoon he found himself at the Chinese restaurant on Guess Road. He had no idea why he was there—that he was looking for more time and love with his family. The whole group was quiet for a while, taking in just how simple and profoundly emotional our relationships with food can be. Usually, the underlying feelings we associate with certain types of foods or meals are so obvious, we don't even pay attention to their likely significance—until a situation like this.

You, too, may enjoy an aha moment on doing the following exercise, which can help you explore your emotion and food connections. You may also benefit from participating in an Overeater's Anonymous group or an Adult Children of Alcoholics group; there is nothing quite like an honest, supportive community in which everyone is seeking his or her truth.

Day 4: An Inventory of Food Flashbacks

Examining your favorite foods and your history and association with eating can be very revealing. We often eat particular foods at certain times or in specific places because we are unconsciously seeking the feelings that we have associated with them in the past. Think of your favorite foods, and respond to the following list of items in your journal. This exploration of your emotional history with certain foods, locations, and situations can be done in confidential support groups at the Rice Diet Program or alone with your journal at home. Give yourself ten to fifteen minutes of quiet, uninterrupted time with your journal. In chapter 2, you began to document your food intake in your *Dieta* Journal. You may want to now circle these foods when you eat them, thus highlighting the foods that you realize you are eating for emotional reasons or motives other than hunger.

Favorite foods:

When and where you eat them:

First memory of eating these foods: when, where, and with whom:

What feelings the foods inspire:

Awakening to Healthier Actions: Louise's Story

One Ricer, Louise, captured the essence of this mind-body-spirit journey in a journalizing class during her first week on the program, after she was notified that her home had been burglarized. Instead of immediately racing home and chasing another drama, she stopped herself. She saw for the first time what she realized was a major pattern in her life: when attempting to take care of herself, she would quickly think that something else deserved her attention more. She had already become aware enough to ask herself some important questions: When I feel like I've been victimized, what do I feel and how do I habitually react? When have I felt this way before, and why am I suddenly hungry and desirous of running? Can I feel these feelings and then choose to take full responsibility for them and the choices I make? Can I delegate to others back home, keep my commitment to my health, and create a win-win situation? Louise got it almost instantaneously; she realized that her food issue was not so much about the food but a deeper worthiness issue. She stopped herself from panicking and rushing home, called her daughter, then enrolled her trusted friends, employees, police, and insurance agent to handle the situation while maintaining her top priority—pursuing her health. In the ensuing weeks, she took advantage of our program's many inner healing paths—yoga, tai chi, meditation, journalizing, and mindfulness eating exercises—using all of her senses. One day she showed up for a journalizing session in which I invited the participants to dialogue with a part of their body they had ignored or divorced. Here is Louise's conversation with her stomach:

Hello, let me reintroduce myself. I am your stomach. You have spent years ignoring me, hating me, being disgusted with me. Do you realize how important I am to you?! But yet, you ignore me, always turning your head away in disgust and disgrace. You treated me as though I was invisible. Interestingly, the more years you ignored me, the more visible I became. I am important in your life. Please reacquaint yourself with me. I am the organ that stores and digests the food you decide to put into your body. I am just doing my job to keep you alive and well. Would you please consider all I do for you and give me the respect and dignity I deserve and long for? I am not the one who dictates what is put into me. It is you, my Dear Master. By placing only healthy, nutritious food into me, soon you will someday be proud to look at me again. And we will both feel the dignity and the same joy we did when we were younger. How about it?! Let us end the alienation saga today. From this day forward, let's align our body and spirit together in synchronicity. I will support your efforts every step of the way. Together, we can co-create the miracle to make your dream come true. Thank you for acknowledging me after all the years of silence. I've been lonely and missed you. If you give me a chance, you'll find that I am your friend and ally. Please learn to love me again. Always remember that what you love, you empower. And what you fear, you empower. And what you empower, you attract.

By the next morning, Louise told me that she had chosen to take full responsibility for committing to her needed weight loss. Louise had begun her journey by asking herself questions she knew the answers to. Through prompt, conscious choices, she learned a very valuable lesson: when she feels like a victim, she can choose to realize it, feel it, and seek her Creative Source of the Universe (whom she knows as God) before proceeding with the best choice for her, rather than reacting out of fear and a victim mentality. Louise learned on a new level that you get to show up for yourself.

Dig Deeper and Uncover the Root of Your Problem

Most of us are aware that if we get really stressed out about something, we often feel the effect in our bodies. Some of us also realize that being overweight, having high blood pressure, or suffering from pain in the neck are related to stress and unprocessed feelings and emotional experiences. It is interesting that many people place certain diseases such as fibromyalgia or drug- and food-addiction disorders in the psychosomatic category, assuming that when individuals suffer from these ailments, "it's all in their heads" or that they are "emotionally out of control." Some may judge these groups of people to be spiritually afflicted with diseases as punishment because of their sinful or destructive choices; then there is also the blameless category, where people are judged to have simply inherited defective genes or been dealt a bad hand that they had no part in creating. Although we can describe and define all sorts of diagnoses and theories for the occurrence of various diseases, the truth is that no one fully knows their causes. Because we are all so uniquely different, how could we totally understand our own diseases—much less someone's whom we barely know? I am sure about one thing, however: remaining stuck in blame and shame does not serve you or others. It harms them instead.

We will all improve our health and our chances of fulfilling our potential if we approach the concept—or the reality—of any disease as an opportunity for growth and development. I've seen hundreds of Ricers experience tremendous healing from this simple yet profound shift in point of view. I, too, have experienced this shift, as a result of my numerous health challenges and healings. In essence, we greatly improve our chances of healing when we look to the root source of our pain—whether that be physical (unhealthy eating habits and inactivity), mental (a negative mind-set, a victim mentality, or a sense of poverty or scarcity), or emotional (unhealthy feelings usually stemming from early pain or trauma, which inspired self-defeating belief systems).

Again, it wasn't until I was healed of a severe crippling joint disorder that I fully realized that my unhealthy, habitual relationship with an emotion—resentment—had disabled me and had also healed me in a deep way.

When strangers first hear of my joint disorder, they often assume that because my mother had numerous types of arthritis, I must have inherited a genetic propensity for having arthritic problems. Yet I now know that I unconsciously contributed to my symptoms of intense joint pain at that time by responding to a cascading series of events with chronic feelings of resentment. During this period of my life, I often awoke with clenched fists, obviously unwilling to release my grip on a situation that I was certainly not in control of, and in ways that were clearly not creating the change I most desired—which was to be free of pain. I underwent nine months of inner healing, which consisted of a steady practice of emotional and spiritual introspection and energy work that included yoga, meditation, journalizing, and a little work with a 12-step Adult Children of Alcoholics group and a psychotherapist. Then I participated in a weekend retreat on emotional healing facilitated by Dr. Waldemar "Wally" Purcell, the most discerning and gifted psychotherapist I have ever had the pleasure of knowing. In one of the afternoon laboratory sessions, during which people shared openly from their hearts, he asked us to complete the assignment described for Day 5 (see the next page). Afterward, Wally asked the group whether anyone cared to participate in a role-playing experience.

With my typical type A, "go for all the healing I can get" approach, I enthusiastically waved my raised arm around. I thought that role-playing sounded like fun. I was very clear that I really wanted, and fully expected, to be totally healed. Well, to summarize this phenomenally amazing and physically, mentally, emotionally, and spiritually transformative experience as succinctly as possible, I will say that I immediately *felt* different. (I will describe the transformative spiritual highlights of this experience in chapter 5.) Although my physical joint pain was still present for another week, I knew on an emotional, intuitive level that my control addiction, or chronic, habitual dependence on the resentment of other controlling people, had forever changed. It was a week later when my physical pain was completely healed. I pray that you will find this exercise as revealing and potentially healing for your particular emotional issues as I did for mine. You are welcome to duplicate the following exercise for your journal or ongoing emotional inventories and explorations.

Day 5: Unpack Your Baggage

The following journalizing exercise is a simple technique for examining the emotional roots of your unease or disease. Create a quiet place when you have ten to fifteen minutes; take a few deep breaths and ask your most troubling issue to surface. Think of the last time you felt the overwhelming hold of a certain emotion or disease, then trace it back to the underlying root. Responding to the statements in the list below will help you in this. Sometimes this is obvious.

For instance, if you have recurring headaches and ask yourself to become conscious of what precedes them, it is often so blatantly simple and clear that it is laughable. *Oh yeah, I only get headaches when my teenager comes home and we fight like cats and dogs.* In other words, when you try to control people and do not produce the results you desire, a headache results. Under *Emotions that are not serving my higher calling* you might write "Frustration and anger when my authority is disregarded." *Situational examples* could include "Unproductive daily fights with teenage son" and "Emotional eating when no one wins." *Plans to Heal* could list options like: "Seek therapist that Sue recommended," "Create more positive interactions such as eating together at my son's favorite restaurant and enjoying his movie choice this weekend," "Research parent-teenage retreats that are focused on such challenges," and "Practice journalizing and meditation instead of emotional eating."

Sometimes, when this is not as obvious, you may benefit by doing this exercise with your most trusted confidante or therapist. Following this exercise with a role-playing therapist who knew how to take me to a deeper level of understanding was what preceded my healing from a supposedly incurable crippling joint disorder.

Show up for your healing by responding to the statements below in your journal.

Emotions that do not serve my higher calling:

Situational examples that precipitate these feelings:

Plans to heal:

Often, I hear Ricers express their amazement that their food obsessions and feelings of hunger are totally gone the first day on the program, but then later they admit that their hunger came back right after their ex-husband called to argue further about the divorce! Yes, we all eat for emotional reasons, and we create a lot of problems for ourselves that we are oblivious to—until we choose to become conscious to them.

The Responsibility Game

The Responsibility Game was introduced to me by Rob Katz, the director of the Legacy Center in Morrisville, North Carolina, where I participated in a leadership training program called the Journey. It is a simple, yet effective way to manage even the most intense emotions and disempowering mind-sets. In a concrete, practical way, it teaches you how to use the law of attraction, a law of physics that is defined as like attracting like. It will teach you this principle by letting you consciously approach your life like a game, which can help you understand that your positive thoughts, feelings, and faith, when intentionally enjoyed simultaneously, can fuel your co-creative abilities to manifest your heart's desires. This practice can greatly help you let go of feelings you may have of being a victim to what happens outside of you.

This tool can make the journey into your emotions fun yet powerful, while not igniting the blame or shame response that many readers may know too well. When Rob coached me during the proposal stage of this book, he introduced me to the Responsibility Game, which is about claiming your power in life. Rob said, "Every time you make a choice that gives you power, you use that power to move ahead toward your goal. It might be a big step or it might be a tiny step, but it's moving forward. Every step ahead earns a point in the game. Every time you allow your feelings to stop you from moving ahead, you've given up your power. Every time you see your situation as hopeless or overwhelming, you miss a step or even take a step backward. Each blocked or backward step costs you a point in the game.

"When you've scored enough points to achieve your goal, you win the game. That is, when you make enough choices to claim your power, and you use it enough times to succeed at your goal, you've won. Celebrate! Do a victory dance! Then you can set your sights on your next goal and play again."

Rob told me about Laura, who was a marketing executive and a mom, raising four kids who included her teenage son Tommy. She worked daily with Tommy, helping him through the typical struggles that teenagers face, until one unforgettable day that changed her life. Laura came home from work to find that Tommy had killed himself. Laura's husband blamed her and filed for divorce. When she moved away to start a new life, her family stopped supporting her and, at times, even refused to talk to her. This is enough to devastate many people, but today Laura is happily remarried and is the director of a teenage leadership program that touches hundreds of lives. How does Laura rise above her circumstances? She plays, and habitually wins, the Responsibility Game.

In every situation in life, you always have choices you can make. Even in the worst of life's tragedies, you still have choices. If nothing else, you can always choose your attitude. Every time you look at a situation as if you have some power over it, you put yourself in the driver's seat of your life. Every time you see your power in a situation, you can take a step forward toward your goals. Conversely, every time you look at a situation as if you have no authority or say in the matter, you have no power.

What is the Responsibility Game? It is a way of looking at the world and a way of living life. The objective of this game is to achieve your goals. By playing the Responsibility Game, you are much more successful at having your life be the way you want it to be. Your game's strategy is determined by the goals you set: you reach your weight and your health goals, you make more money, and/or the quality of your relationships go up . . . whatever you have prioritized as your game's goals. The game is an easy yet potent way to make your life turn out the way you want it to.

Like any game, the Responsibility Game has points to score, it has a way to win, and it has some rules to follow. To earn points in this game, you make choices that put you in control of your life. A responsibility choice is choosing a viewpoint about what's happening that gives you power to affect the situation, rather than feel powerless about it. You look at what's happening around you and decide how you feel about it. What will be your attitude about it? "My kids are rambunctious today—I'm thrilled they are so healthy and vibrant." "My kids are rambunctious today—they are going to drive me crazy!" Once you are conscious of your thoughts and feelings, you can enjoy them, be angered by them, or choose to shift your attitude.

Laura could have easily seen herself as powerless after the death of her son, her divorce, and her family's response. At times, her feelings were so strong that she was overwhelmed by them. Playing the Responsibility Game, however, she knew that her goals were to provide a safe and loving environment for her family and to save other teens before they committed suicide. Every day she made choices. Some days she scored many points, and the children she worked with received all of her love and caring. Other days she didn't score many points. Over time, by staying focused on her goals, not only did she score enough points to heal and expand her family, but she also created a position where she may prevent her tragedy from happening to others.

It is a very challenging and exciting game to be alert and recognize your responsibility to be truly aware of your present thoughts and feelings; you can cultivate the mindfulness to assess whether you want to continue to create from that paradigm or shift to a stand that positively supports the outcome you want. My team for the Legacy Center Journey was called NC73B, and our motto was "Shift happens." And it does! You can choose to take full responsibility for steering your emotional rudders, or you can waste a lot of potentially creative time being stuck on events or actions whose emotions you don't want to feel. This invitation to "shift from self-defeating emotional states to empowering ones" is not meant to encourage you to minimize your emotional processing of pain or suffering, which can be powerful teachers, but to remember that you don't have to camp out there or become frozen with inertia. When you become an active player in the Responsibility Game, you develop a habit of consciously choosing to perceive everything as an opportunity to win your heart's desire and maximize your life's potential.

The Responsibility Game is a way of looking at the world and approaching your life as if you can make a difference in how it evolves. You either think you are responsible for creating the life goals you have, or you don't and thus are willing to accept the victim role in your life. You may be saying, "Yeah, this is true most of the time, *but* what about . . . blah, blah, blah?" I don't want to hear your *but* story; it will not serve you in actualizing your goals or the life that you want. I am inviting you to enter a paradigm shift in consciousness, which is nothing more than a shift, or change, in your way of perceiving the world and your power in co-creating the world. Those who have made the greatest shifts in their consciousness usually have done so due to a compelling reason or a sense that it is important for them to do so. This is why it may often seem easier if you seek change during a life crisis, such as a divorce, a family death, or a heart attack, but you don't have to wait for a big Mack truck to hit you!

Day 6: Responsibility Game Jump-Start

Act as if you are responsible for everything that happens in your life, in a quiet place, with journal in hand, for fifteen to twenty paradigm-shifting minutes. Two key qualities for successful change and paradigm shifts are having a clear idea of what you want and being committed to following the goal through to completion. Prime your paradigm shift by developing clarity of heart about what your goals really are and how achieving them will look, feel, smell, taste, and sound. Let go of any limiting thoughts. You may want to keep score in your journal's margin, chalking up a point every time you release a thought that negatively affects the pursuit of your goal. Remember that shifting paradigms and expanding one's consciousness involve taking risks, as does any significant growth or change, so don't forget that any fall or slip gets to be followed by scoring more points when you get up again!

I hear Dr. Kempner chant, "It's not the intensity of the great passion but the duration of the great passion that makes a great man (and woman) great!" Inspire all of your senses to support you in your conscious pursuit of your goals and the life that you want. And keep getting up for the next inning of play!

Use Music to Shift Your Health Consciousness

One day my brother, Digger, called me as he was driving down the road, rocking out to his latest Austin, Texas, music discovery. He said, "Kitty, if you are going to be writing a book about how to create paradigm shifts, describing ways to help shift our minds and hearts into more positive directions, you've got to include music. There is no faster way for me to move from a complete funk, to flying high, than by popping in the right rock 'n' roll!" I knew that music certainly did this for me, and this conversation set me off on a journey to learn more about it.

I began to incorporate music into our program's offering of healing tools after I read of the most recent scientific research that substantiated music's health benefits. The influence of music is boundless; think about its role in your life. Music can excite; it can relax; and it can transport, carrying us from the present to some point in the past. A song can produce a flood of memories. Music's power in the human experience is not a new phenomenon. In fact, early humans believed that music could free the body of evil spirits. Prominent scholars throughout history—Plato, Pythagoras, Aristotle, and Al-Farabi (known as Alpharabius in Europe)—have recognized the restorative effects of music. More recently, music has been shown to elicit a therapeutic relaxation response in the body, leading to multiple health benefits.

According to early research in this area, stress and relaxation responses are mutually exclusive events. Music may act as a distraction or a diversion from stressful stimuli, or it may act directly on the autonomic nervous system. When the relaxation response occurs, the stress response is interrupted and anxiety levels decrease. By mediating the response of the parasympathetic division of the nervous system, relaxing music exerts a protective effect on the heart. As the activity of the parasympathetic nervous system increases, stress levels in the body decrease. Heart rate, blood pressure, and myocardial oxygen requirements also decrease. These responses ultimately have a positive effect on heart health. Multiple research studies have shown that music therapy improves patient outcomes after a heart attack.

The use of music as a therapeutic healing method is gaining in popularity, as evidenced by the growing body of relevant research. In addition to benefiting heart patients, music therapy has been used to help terminally ill patients decrease depressive symptoms, lessen social isolation, and increase communication, self-expression, and relaxation.

As I combed the latest research on the health benefits of music, it became clear that music, in general, is good for you. Relaxation music was the primary type that was researched, but self-selected music was also found to be beneficial, and even more so when you actively sang or played an instrument. So, as you read about the following research studies, be mindful of what music you enjoy, and be ready to jot down some songs or genres that you may want to add to your music library. Songs that go from your head to your heart will stimulate all of the forms of positivity that Dr. Barbara Fredrickson, a professor of psychology and the principal investigator of the Positive Emotions and Psychophysiology Laboratory at the University of North Carolina–Chapel Hill, described in her recent book *Positivity: Groundbreaking Research Reveals How to Embrace the Hidden Strength of Positive Emotions, Overcome Negativity, and Thrive*: joy, gratitude, serenity, interest, hope, pride, amusement, inspiration, awe, and love. So feed your soul what it most desires; a heartfelt song, played or belted out passionately, can truly satisfy your emotional hunger.

The University of Frankfurt in Germany found that singing enhanced the immune systems of singers. On completion of performing Mozart's *Requiem*, members of the choir had higher levels of immunoglobulin A; listeners experienced lower levels of cortisol, a classic relaxation response. Choir singing was also found to promote improved lung capacity, higher energy levels, relief from asthma, better posture, a positive mood, and enhanced feelings of relaxation and confidence. Gene D. Cohen, the director of the Center on Aging, Health, and Humanities at George Washington University, led research on creativity and aging among a choral group of senior citizens. The results surprised even the researchers. Because the average age of the seniors was eighty, some decline in health was expected, rather than the actual improvement in health that directly related to their participation in the arts. The groups involved in the arts reported fewer doctor visits, eyesight problems, and falls, as well as less depression and need for medication. Researcher Robert Beck, at the University of California–Irvine, administered a saliva test to choir members and found increased levels of immunity-building proteins. These proteins increased 150 percent during a rehearsal and 240 percent during a performance, and increases occurred over a two- to three-hour period.

Dr. Diane Austin, a vocal psychotherapist in private practice, wrote about the benefits of singing: "Singing facilitates deep breathing. . . . Deep breathing slows the heart rate and calms the nervous system, stilling the mind and body." She also noted that singing produces vibrations in the body much like an internal massage, vibrations that can help release blocks in the body and allow for a more vital flow of energy.

The benefits of listening to, moving to, or creating music or song can be enjoyed alone or with a choir. Findings suggest, and your common sense will concur, that the music you listened to when you were seventeen to twenty-one years of age will have the greatest effect for you. Not only are there more neurological pathways that were developed during those years from replaying these songs, they hold significantly more emotional connections for you, which can assist you in shifting your mood from frustration (and wanting to numb out with your food or drug of choice) to empowerment, pleasure, and wanting to go after your life again. It makes no difference whether you can carry a tune or not; benefits have been found with humming; lip trills; chanting a specific word or phrase ("let it be" or "I can't get no satisfaction"); singing inspiring songs that encourage joy, peace, and enthusiasm to persevere and take your life on as if it really matters; and singing along with a singer whose voice represents a quality and a way of being that you wish to embody (tender, strong, grounded, resurrected).

Plugging into a positive sound is a powerful pathway to healing that will especially appeal to people who are auditory learners, those who already appreciate music, and others who are in need of "changing the channel" from depressing news or talk radio to affirming and empowering music that will elevate them throughout the day. Yet incorporating music into my groups at the Rice Diet Program has taught me that you can never predict who will best respond to this sensory approach.

After giving participants a quantum physics description of the power of consciously thinking, feeling, and intending what one desires, I often facilitate groups in which I have them meditate, then journalize on what comes up for them while empowering music is played. Not only does the listening modality approach and reach us from a new sense (hearing), thus affirming the message to a different set of neurons, its empowering words can move the mental (thought) energy to the heart's center. When we truly comprehend the research that shows that the heart's magnetic field is approximately five thousand times stronger than the field produced by the brain, we further appreciate the techniques that move head knowledge to our hearts. As HeartMath practitioners' and many quantum physicists', neurophysiologists', and neuropsychologists' research now shows, when a thought becomes a feeling, it can shift our belief system and then allow our desired results to manifest.

One day I led a group of Ricers into a meditation as I played the song "I Believe I Can Fly." Such commanding, echoing, and crescendoing words, with an equally compelling melody, can often inspire the most defeated of souls into opening up to their truth. I then asked the participants to write about whatever had come to their minds and hearts. After the session, a Ricer, who had previously admitted her strong analytical and critical, left-brained tendencies, shared her amazement that she had immediately become in touch with feelings that she did not realize were within her capacity to enjoy or even optimistically consider. She wrote that she desired "a committed relationship that would allow her to share her life to its fullest, with companionship and love." After the group had dispersed, she revealed that following her physically abusive husband's death, she had avoided any type of committed relationship like the plague. Her memories were so painful that for fifteen years after her husband's death, whenever she was under stress, she had nightmares that he was still alive and was returning, and she would have to live with him again. During standard psychotherapy, she was led to confront and forgive him, and the nightmares ceased. Yet the ability to allow any man into her life was not yet possible. This combination of mediums for right-brain nourishment was what she needed to reveal to herself that given she could do anything she wanted, she really could believe and accept that a man could become a part of her life, one whom she could share everything with—a possibility that she had not allowed herself to entertain for more than thirty years!

This was not magic; we all have much wisdom within that will benefit our journey when we seek answers from places deeper than our left, analytical brains. And music continues to inspire our participants into experiencing paradigm shifts in consciousness, which allows this innate wisdom to become part of their waking awareness.

Day 7: Moving Your Head and Heart with Music

In this present moment, act as if you could be part of co-creating anything you want in your life. Remove your blinders and any veil limiting your vision; relax the critical mind, and encourage the right brain and the creative, intuitive truth within. You may want to buy the *Healing at the Roots: Songs of Renewal* CD that was produced to accompany this book, or download some head- and heart-opening music to your mp3 player or hard drive. Some tried-and-true ones we use here at the program are "I Believe I Can Fly" (R. Kelly), "It's in Everyone of Us" (David Pomerantz), "You Raise Me Up" (Josh Groban), and "Be Ye Glad" (Michael Kelly Blanchard). Any song that stimulates your head and heart to expand is helpful.

Julee Glaub Weems and her husband, Mark Weems, a duo known as Little Windows, have collaborated with me to produce *Healing at the Roots*, inspired and appropriately named to comple-ment this book. It is full of heart-, head-, and spirit-connecting traditional Celtic and American music. Check it out at www .ricedietstore.com or www.littlewindows.net. Purchasing this CD from either site is recommended for those interested in reading the liner notes, background information, and song lyrics, which will further help you to realize the full potential of inviting all of your senses to the healing experience.

After listening to an inspiring song or two, start to journalize on whatever comes to your mind. Depending on your musical choices and your present internal emotional state, you may choose to write on the top five things that you most want in your life. If that is the case, "I Believe I Can Fly" will certainly inspire and encourage you. On the other hand, you may be in the midst of processing grief, sorrow, loneliness, or loss and need your hope deepened and enriched by listening to Little Windows' "Queen of the Night," "Blue Hills of Why," and "Healer of My Soul." Tune into yourself and the music that can most help you tap into your emotional need for healing.

Music and Its Effect on Life

Music correlates with life and deepens your life experience in many ways, some yet to be discovered. A few interesting observations from Daniel J. Levitin in *This Is Your Brain on Music: The Science of a Human Obsession* include his thoughts on melody and pitch, among others. He described melody as music that is based on a scale, such as when we would say that the melody is in the key of C. He elaborates that this means that the melody has a momentum to return to the note C; it will not necessarily end on the note C but will have C as the most prominent and focal note of the overall piece. Although notes may temporarily be used outside of the C major scale, "like a quick edit in a movie to a parallel scene or a flashback, in which we know that a return to the main plotline is imminent and inevitable," we are confident in our soul that the composer will be taking us home. When I read his description on melody, I was moved by how much the melody of music reflects our perspective on life, our paradigms, and how we expect our future to reflect our past—whether we realize it or not. For instance, if we hear a song in the key of C, we expect variations but are most comfortable if it stays or ends near C, just as if we have habitually been raised in a positive family, surrounded by empowering expectations, we are much more likely to anticipate a future that flourishes and expands, than is someone who was raised with negative influences and whose early life experiences set up painfully limited intentions. But the good news is that positivity can be developed and nurtured to grow; the new research on music's benefits is significant and substantial.

Sandra's Story

One of the most exciting breakthroughs that I've seen in a Ricer this year was in Sandra, who had participated numerous times before but returned with a new sense of readiness. The freedom expressed in her eyes now reflects her story, as do her following words.

My first visit to the Rice Diet Program was in 1999. From the start, I realized that for me, this was much more than a diet. It was a spiritual journey into my soul, as well as how to lose weight and rev up my physical exercise. The sense of community, the classes in yoga, journalizing, the doctors' care and attention, and the education given were priceless. Everything that was offered stirred in me the feeling that perhaps I could regain control of my life and body, something I had clearly lost in the preceding fifteen years.

At the same time, I started attending Dr. Rosati's meditation class. Meditation is known to change the hormones in the "feel good" part of the brain, which can go a long way in alleviating some addictive compulsions when combined with other factors. This understanding sang to me, and seeds of a passion to help people and myself were planted within me. I survived divorce, dysfunctional family life, and financial reversals. Here was always a place I could come to replenish and heal.

This year I decided that maintenance of over two hundred pounds had not served me well, and it was time to get the job done and pursue my distant dream. And now came my epiphany: for the first time, I returned to the Rice House weighing less than when I left! I attended one of Kitty's classes on all the interpersonal aspects of the Rice *dieta*. She played a YouTube bite of Wintley Phipps singing a magnificent rendition of "Amazing Grace." My first reaction was, "Wow, that is one of my favorite songs," and then my mind zoomed to the movie *Amazing Grace* and how it impacted me—to the possibility that one person could make a difference when driven with passion and deliberation.

Later that day, I was in a store and over the sound system I heard the song "Amazing Grace." The next day, I was coming back to my room after a nice walk, and just to relax a bit,

I sat down and turned on *Oprah*—and Il Divo was singing "Amazing Grace"! That evening I was at the movies with a friend, and I told her of my experience and asked if something was going on. The movie was *The Secret Life of Bees*, and in the middle was, of course, "Amazing Grace." I was totally confused and blown away. I felt it was way past coincidence. I called one of my daughters and recounted this story, and she said, "Maybe you are supposed to make a difference!" I hope I can one day realize my dream and make that difference for others.

You may be sitting there thinking that Sandra's story sounds painfully like yours, but you feel that your life is still largely disabled by your emotional baggage. You may be feeling better since you have already vastly improved your diet and exercise habits, have started journalizing, and have even actively participated in the experiential challenges that have begun to open your mind to new possibilities, but you are still unsettled by how your feelings can unpredictably carry you away like a tsunami. Don't worry, feeling your emotions can be a terrifying experience if you haven't done so in a few decades, and you may feel worse before you feel better, but the good news is, you will feel better, and any pain will be worth the upcoming rewards of unloading your emotional baggage!

Day 8: Listen to the Song of Life

My musician friend Julee shared this amazing story about the palliative and healing effect of music. Julee and her husband, Mark, travel around the world singing and teaching professionally (learn about them at www.littlewindows.net). They often give workshops on the power of traditional song and tell stories about its timeless and mysterious nature. Traditional song has connections to a larger picture of generations past and songs that have been passed down from family to family. Traditional song comes out of a deep sense of community, from gatherings on mountain porches to singers around a turf fire in Ireland. As Julee recalled,

One of the stories that carries one of strongest imprints would be my encounter with Peg Perry and her sister Katharine Hepburn. I was at a crossroads in my life. I had left my home in North Carolina to take a year to figure out whether I was to do music or teach full time. I had tried my hand and heart at teaching in a classroom but quickly knew that was not for me. I knew I wanted to continue teaching in some capacity and also sensed a strong calling to music. Yet there was great turmoil in my soul, as I had some horrible encounters with a musician I had been working with who was focused on money, ego, and dishonesty. I remember going out in my hay field in Connecticut one night, looking up at the stars, and acknowledging that "I quit" if music was going to be like this . . . working with folks whom I could not relate to, whose motive and focus seemed to be so different from mine.

Soon after my declaration, the phone rang inside my wee cabin in the woods. It was Peg, my neighbor and older friend, who had become a grandmother figure in my life. She was inviting me to accompany her on her weekly visit to see her sister Katharine down at the shore, "And bring your guitar." Several days later, we turned into a long, winding driveway and first met a large sign shooing away any trespassers; drove up to the door, where we were warmly greeted by Katharine's caretaker; delivered Peg's weekly homemade bread; and walked into a beautiful old New England beach house, museumlike and filled with photos of Katharine and Spencer in their prime. We went into the living room, where Katharine sat in a big ole chair overlooking the sea beside the fireplace, ornamented with a sign, which read "Listen to the Song of Life."

That day opened up my ears and heart to listen more intuitively to the song of life. As I wrestled with my own thoughts and feelings, which widely ranged from the fact that I was visiting an icon, a woman who had done more for our world of movies and entertainment than about anyone I could think of . . . yet here she was, frail, deaf, and alone in a big ole house by the sea. Peg introduced us, and with her Katie Hepburn head-shaking way she said, "Your hair is very curly."

She was dear and welcomed me warmly. After a little lunch, Peg asked me to get out my guitar. I sang her several Irish songs, and Katharine began to talk about her memories of Ireland with Spencer's relations, stories of the beach at Old Saybrook, and requests for more songs. Her feet moved to and fro as if she were dancing in her chair. Several times I had to stop and wipe her tears with a tissue in between verses, and then we shared laughter together as well. It was soon time for her nap, and we got back in the car to travel an hour and a bit home. Peg immediately said, "That was charming," in her Hepburn family way and proceeded to tell me that her sister had not spoken or conversed like that in years. The music had released her heart, her memories, and even her speech. It was that day that I realized I was to sing for the rest of my life.

Whether you have the Irish life experience that Kate had, the fun memories of the Fiddler's Convention that I do, or never even heard traditional Scots-Irish or Appalachian Old Time music, most people are moved by it. Regardless of your gene pool, I would encourage you to explore this and other genres outside of your favorite golden oldies. Traditional music has survived this long because it can go straight to our core, and it is worth exploring. Whether it is Little Windows' nature-inspiring "I Wandered By a Brookside" or "Let the Life I Lead," which awakens and renews your desire to live on purpose, these traditional songs will open you to a healing of the heart. Traditional singers pass on what was known earlier, yet their personal experiences of their everyday struggles and celebrations with family, work, and God still speak to us deeply because much of what is important to us humans does not really change much. There seems to be a mythic quality to these old songs, which may represent a way of life and community to which many of us are unconsciously drawn. These songs were sung while people milked cows, fed babies, gathered flowers, worked the land, and

visited neighbors. Amid the complexity of our modern lives, perhaps we find healing in the melodies and the lyrics that have stood
the test of time for hundreds of years.

When I first started to use music with my meditation and journalizing sessions, I played only empowering, affirming songs, but
more and more I recognized the healing that is inherent in songs
of suffering as well. I have come to appreciate that there is a good
reason for the large percentage of these darker songs that have survived to form the official canon of traditional song; by entering into
them, a personal healing is available. Thank you, Mark and Julee,
for expanding my repertoire for healing!

Although we all have probably known on some level that music
is empowering and can shift us from feeling depressed and disabled
faster than just about anything we can think of, it is also inspiring
to know that the research supporting this activity is substantial.
And science is always more satisfying and affirming when coupled
with a real-life resurrection story. Just imagining Julee's angelic
voice prompting a socially isolated, nearly deaf and dying Katharine
Hepburn to move her feet and ask for more songs makes me very
happy and ever more convinced that music can help us all experience
more during our lives. It is freeing to know that any music you like
to hear will be health promoting, so surround yourself with sound!
Rather than checking out from a stressful workday with aggressive
or valueless television programming and unconscious consumption
of processed foods, why not pocket your mp3 player, downloaded
with your favorite songs, throw on your sneakers, and walk the dog,
for a free, calorie-burning, mood-uplifting, health-promoting good
time? Improving your mood and losing weight while you jam to your
top tunes is a winning combination for creating weight loss that is
sustainable.

Becoming Free of Difficult Emotions

The power of your body to process emotion and let go of difficult
or traumatic emotional experiences can often be expedited and

realized even more dramatically through a practice known as emotional freedom technique (EFT). A few years ago, Dr. Larry Burk, a radiologist and a dear and respected friend, was the director of education at the Duke Center for Integrative Medicine, responsible for organizing the people involved in complementary medicine. He often invited me to speak to Duke's medical students, and I invited him to come over with his students to see how we at the Rice Diet Program prevent and reverse chronic disease, with an emphasis on empowering the patient. For the last seven years, he has taught and practiced EFT, a self-healing method that is being taught to thousands of people all around the world. It was first developed by Gary Craig, a Stanford University–trained engineer, who describes this method as a "needle-free version of acupuncture that is based on new discoveries regarding the connection between your body's subtle energies, your emotions and your health." A summary of this method is available for free at www.emofree.com. Although this is a relatively new therapy, you will quickly note from reading the information on this Web site and the references in the back of this book that substantial and impressive research results have been accumulating since 2003.

This very simple and safe approach to dealing with chronic pain, past emotional traumas, and current anxieties is also very useful for weight loss and is especially helpful in dealing with food cravings. It involves self-tapping on acupuncture meridian points while repeating short statements about a particular emotional experience or belief. Tapping on the acupoints in this fashion deletes the body memory of the issue that is connected to the cognitive memory, allowing anxiety to be replaced by emotional freedom.

In one example, a fifty-year-old overweight woman complained that she craved chocolate so much that she had to eat a large candy bar every day to calm her nerves. She used EFT to give up this addiction by starting with the phrase "Even though I crave chocolate when I am anxious, I deeply and completely accept myself." After doing the EFT tapping for ten minutes, she returned a month later to report that her freezer full of chocolate bars had not been touched since the last visit, and she had lost ten pounds.

Eight different acupoints are used during EFT, beginning on top of the head, then down the face, on the collarbone, and finally under the armpit (see the illustration below). Once you learn where they are, the process takes only a few minutes. You tap seven times on each of the acupoints with your index and middle fingers while repeating your phrases shortened, such as, "I overeat when I am anxious" or "I overeat when I am bored." After tapping down each side of your body, you report your subjective units of distress before and after tapping on a scale of 0 to 10, with 0 being no distress and 10 being the worst you can imagine. Some issues go to 0 and disappear immediately after the tapping, never to return, especially those relating to situations from the past. Others take some persistence, particularly when they relate to ongoing stressful situations. EFT can be repeated as often as needed, and there are no adverse side effects. There is no catharsis or drama. The most that people

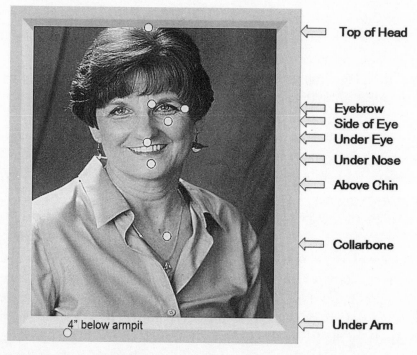

The location of acupoints used during EFT.

usually experience is a few tears related to difficult subjects that they are tapping about, but that quickly shifts to feelings of relief.

Larry now follows this first series of tapping with the negative phrases, on both sides of your body, with three more series of tapping the negative phrases and alternating them with positive phrases, such as "When I am anxious, I take a walk" and "When I am bored, I tap and laugh, thinking this crazy stuff might work!" When he does this introductory session of EFT at the Rice Diet Program, we are often laughing because at first it seems so bizarre and hocus-pocus, but when we experience and then hear the results it can create, we keep tapping!

One of the most impressive EFT healings I've personally witnessed was a woman at the Rice Diet Program who had an intense phobia of insects, especially cockroaches. Her phobia so controlled her life that she would actually have to leave her home if she even saw a cockroach. Because she lived in a semitropical climate, this was very disruptive to her life. I heard her story and tapped with her for the hourlong session. Then I saw her again six months later when she returned to report to Larry in the EFT class that after that one session, she had gone home and frankly forgotten about the phobia! It was only after her husband and her son saw her pick up a dead cockroach and throw it outside, and they expressed amazement at her lack of fear, that she realized she had even previously had that phobia! This was incredibly convincing, because the woman is very understated, and I don't believe she made this up. As I had noticed only slight shifts in my thinking after practicing EFT, it was only after her experience that I began to get excited about its potential. EFT research is growing, and its efficacy is most impressive in helping people with phobias and post-traumatic stress disorders.

Day 9: Emotional Freedom Technique

"The real drivers in weight-loss cases are emotional issues such as self-worth and anxiety," explains Gary Craig. "Until these emotions are properly resolved, willpower will take a backseat and the need for 'comfort foods' will win out every time."

New York City therapist Carol Look agrees. "When you use sugar or overeating as a way to numb your feelings," says Dr. Look, "no diet in the world can help you. Even the latest surgery does nothing to correct underlying emotional imbalances that trigger overeating. EFT doesn't focus on calorie restriction. Instead, it targets emotions that lead to immediate cravings, hunger pangs, and poor eating habits, such as emotions triggered by daily stress, issues from the past, a family history of obesity, limiting beliefs about one's ability to lose weight, fear of the future, and other factors that trigger binges."

EFT addresses these issues by combining focused thought with gentle fingertip tapping on key acupressure points. Dr. Look and other EFT practitioners worldwide report a 50 to 80 percent success rate for those who tap for weight loss, and the results, especially for specific cravings, are often immediate.

Do it yourself, and judge by the results.

Choose an emotional problem or an undesirable symptom to test your hand at your first EFT tapping experiment. Go to www.emofree.com and read the wealth of information that the founder, Gary Craig, has offered to the world for free. Do at least one session per day for a week, and note in your journal any changes that you experience. If you have a serious overeating disorder, do your best to commit to his suggestion of undertaking frequent EFT treatments for a few weeks. With no adverse side effects and positive responses probable, it is a challenge worth taking!

Abundantly Creating the Health and the Life You Want

To fully heal your heart, you need to believe that true health is yours. Health is about seeking abundance, rather than scarcity. Health is about choosing to embrace positive feelings, rather than getting mired down by negative emotions. In the next chapter, you will turn to the power of your mind to gain access to the limitless joy of true health. But in order to do that, you need to be ready for a shift in perspective—from a view that is limiting to one that is limitless. Often, this change in perspective requires a big paradigm shift, an intense and ongoing awakening that expands and evolves your "come from" to be one in which everyone gets to grow and win.

One of the most immediate ways I experienced a paradigm shift that gave me a lifetime belief in my own power to co-create the life I desire was through a weekend course I participated in at the Legacy Center in Morrisville, North Carolina. This particular weekend intensive was called "The Abundance and Prosperity Workshop."

During that weekend, participants really grew to understand how giving with no strings attached was connected with receiving abundantly, versus taking or being tightly bound to the scarcity mentality. When you give to get or are expecting a return, it just doesn't work! We also learned that there are many ways to be out-flowing: smile, go for a walk, check in with yourself or others, be honest, and persist for "the duration of the great passion."

The word *enthusiasm* comes from the Greek words *en* and *theos* that literally translate to "the God within." Enthusiasm is a giving type of energy. It is not a thing to do; it is a "come from," a way of being. Enthusiasm is an expression of abundance. When you bring yourself into enthusiasm, you create abundance. You can create enthusiasm by choosing to be it. You have the power and the choice to bring an enthusiastic experience to any event and to learn to outlast the no's to maintain your enthusiasm.

The book *Flow: The Psychology of Optimal Experience* by Mihaly Csikszentmihalyi includes results from research on people who were asked when they had felt most "alive" in their lives. The people did not describe a beautiful island vacation or relaxing times in the sun but reported that they felt most alive when they were engaged in something big; when they were in the middle of something that they were passionate about, that was making a difference for someone else or the world.

Another word I like to use with Ricers is *wu-wei*, which means plugging into the flow: positive acceptance that you are part of the creative source of the Universe, or all one. It is a state of empowerment, of unlimited abundance. On the other hand, *trishna* means a resistance to the flow, or resisting what is. It includes all negative and limiting thoughts and reflects a state of victimhood and scarcity. A "choice" opens possibilities; a "decision" closes possibilities. After feeling the difference implied in these words, I now say "choose," rather than "decide." To decide is to kill off other choices, and I choose not to suggest a loss of freedom or opportunities. Obviously, positive thinking consistently or habitually requires a moment-to-moment awareness and a choice to do so. And persistence is continually embracing (or surrendering to) a choice you've already made.

Day 10: Create Abundance, Past and Future

One of the experientials I facilitate with Ricers allows them a real-life experience of practicing how to express their enthusiasm, with a partner who listens supportively versus one who negates any possibility they will succeed. It is a very revealing exercise, which you could practice at home with another willing friend.

My game rules involve two people with twenty-four to thirty minutes to share; having a third person to be the timekeeper and facilitator is optimal but not required. You could use a timer to assist you in staying focused on the exercise, rather than on the time. The person sharing gets an opportunity to express his or her enthusiasm for certain goals for the upcoming year (for successful weight loss and all accompanying plans to support this effort, such as specific weight-loss goals, with definitive time frames stated and detailing exercise commitment, cooking agenda, and other creative ways the person will succeed with his or her mission) and exaggerates this passion through body language as well as with words.

You want to think *big*? Take off your blinders and expand your vision on how you will accomplish this goal and *how that feels*. It is easiest to really claim this much confidence and enthusiasm if you speak in the first person and present tense; express yourself as if you are actually standing there one year from today; for instance, "I knew last year when I claimed my year's weight-loss goal of fifty pounds that I would achieve it! I am so thrilled that you are here a year later to celebrate my accomplishments. Remember how I planned to _____, and I did it!" The person sharing will do so for two and a half minutes. Don't worry, the time will fly by; let loose and have some fun with this!

The other person will simply listen supportively. This means mouth closed, ears open, eyes encouraging, and no free advice—the listener should simply be there to hear the friend's goals outlined and the specific details of how he or she will accomplish them.

After two and a half minutes, the listener gets one minute to retell or synthesize what he or she heard; then the original person who initially shared gets thirty seconds to edit or add to the listener's recap.

The exact same experience will be repeated again for two and a half minutes, with the exception that the listener will now repeatedly interrupt with doubting, negative comments. Although this is difficult for some people to hear as they share their passionate, enthusiastically expressed goals, it does give them an opportunity to know what it will feel like when they get home to a world that will not consistently agree with and affirm their best intentions. This time, the person who was attempting to share his or her goals gets a minute to share what it felt like to be interrupted and negated, then the listener has thirty seconds to assure the person that he or she did not enjoy being that negative!

Be sure to end this dyad (exchange between two) with the original person again sharing, for two and a half minutes, his or her enthusiasm for the abundance he or she will have succeeded at co-creating (by a year from today). Have this final role-play exemplify all of the enthusiasm and passion one can express. Again, the listener will take a minute to affirm his or her success and share in the joy that results from being a part of someone's really making a difference in the world. The initial person who shared may again have thirty seconds to add whatever thoughts and feelings have come up.

Then, of course, the same instruction will apply for the second person sharing for two and a half minutes, then listening to what the listener heard for a minute, then having thirty seconds to correct or revise; then repeating it again while the listener interrupts with negative thoughts and attempts to undermine the second person's *wu-wei* with as much *trishna* as is appropriate, and the second individual sharing how this feels. Finally, be sure to have the third role-play crescendo with more abundance and enthusiasm than you have ever mustered up. Think, feel, and be *big*!

All of the groups that I have led through this exercise have been amazed at how different the experience is when we are standing in a state of empowerment, feeling that sense of unlimited abundance, versus the feeling we can get if we surrender to the other's negative comments and doubts.

Samurai warriors were so awesome and legendary in part due to the fact that they faced and accepted death before each battle. This allowed them to war "full on," as if nothing else mattered. It triggered them into *wu-wei*, a place of unlimited potential, a "come from" with no scarcity or fear. Living life having truly faced death can be very liberating and empowering; it can create a *wu-wei* shift into the abundant potential that we all are and all have . . . whether we are Samurai warriors or any human beings who are committed to stand as a source to create a transformed world.

Once you are done, journalize on how you were being in your past when you abundantly created a desired relationship or event. Since giving generously leads to an abundant and prosperous life, how would you need to be in order to have the people and the missions in your life win big during this next year?

The HeartMath Solution

At the Rice Diet Program, we have included specific meditation techniques that align the head and the heart to further heal the heart, including tools advanced by HeartMath Solution research. These data document how if you imagine inhaling into the heart and exhaling from the solar plexus and then recall a positive feeling, such as a feeling of appreciation, of care for someone or for a pet or a place, you will achieve coherence. Because coherence literally shifts your energy from your brain to your heart, which has forty to sixty times more amplitude than that of the brain and a magnetic field approximately five thousand times stronger than the field produced by the brain—get ready for some previously unrealized dreams to bear fruit! For those who are ready to actualize certain intentions and enjoy the resulting paradigm shifts and healing, these exercises can align your head with your heart; they will be well worth the small amount of time that is required for you to practice. This meditation technique reminds me a bit of the loving-kindness meditation practice, in that loving feelings are brought to your heart, energizing this power-packed region. As HeartMath Solution research, publications, and product lines are more directed to serving those in the business world, this approach may appeal to people who like gadgets and gizmos for instant feedback.

Day 11: Your Dream Monologue

Journalize a dream monologue of what you want in your life in five years, three years, one year, six months, and three months. The only limits are your self-imposed ones, so let your imagination run wild! This journalizing assignment was one of the keys to this book's manifesting now rather than later; my three-month expressive writing response really focused my attention on the reality that if this book was going to be published within three years and the musical CD produced within one year, then significant actions were required of me within three months. There is no time like the present moment to harness your heart's desire!

4

Empowering Your Mind

*Our destiny changes with our thoughts; we shall become
what we wish to become, do what we wish to do, when our
habitual thoughts correspond with our desires.*
—Orison Swett Marsden

Your Trigger for Change

There is no one reason that people are inspired to change. For some, it's a health event—a heart attack, a diagnosis, or the death of someone they love. For others, it's more internal or emotional, such as a divorce, the loss of a job or financial security, or any ego-stripping, soul-searching impetus. But that doesn't mean you need a life crisis to make a transformative change in the way you live your life. Many people have expressed to me an inner desire to know who they are, a gnawing hunger to heighten the awareness of their innate ability to harness and co-create the changes they desire in themselves and in the world. The bottom line in your making any successful and lasting change is when your motivation for change weds with a sense of responsibility for yourself. When you are finally ready to accept responsibility for your health, for actualizing your true purpose, when you are finally ready to give up the excuses and stop blaming others or situations beyond your control for what you think you cannot do or accomplish, and you act—you take some physical steps toward your goal—then shift happens!

In my experience, your health is one of the easiest ways you can experience and come to know this creative, healing potential within you. Your health at one level is physical, but when you dig deeper and begin to examine your thoughts related to health, weight, food, and habits and attitudes about food and eating, then you take the next step—you empower your heart and mind. Any disease or challenging life experience can offer you this opportunity to take responsibility for your life, to participate in your healing or co-create any desired change that you choose to pursue. Our human ability to think and the power that our thoughts, feelings, and beliefs have in contributing to our upcoming future have recently received significant attention from quantum physicists and neurophysiologists. And, of course, for centuries, this subject has been explored by religious scholars.

However you wrap your head around the truth, it's good news! The next step in your journey toward attaining true health is examining your thoughts, your behavior patterns, and your overall mindset in order to further clarify what you want and heal any habitual, negative and limiting beliefs that create obstacles to achieving your true desires. You may have negative attitudes about your body or frequent thoughts of your past failures at weight loss. You may also indulge in unconscious behaviors that trigger overeating, such as drinking too much alcohol, skipping meals, or restricting and then bingeing. Or you may chronically entertain thoughts, attitudes, and beliefs that simply aren't true, such as "This is all I should expect in terms of weight-loss success or a career, given my gene pool, track record, or self-assessed opinion of unworthiness."

Yet when you really digest the holistic truth that you are not only what you eat and feel, but also what you think, you can focus on the awareness that is within you, rather than on the *trishna*, or your self-defeating debates or disempowering inner dialogues. With this awareness, you will be co-creating your health. This takes a paradigm shift. Please relax and let go of your attachment to the idea that this process is difficult. We all come into this world with the natural ability to think about what we need and want and thereby release the creative energy to manifest the gifts and talents for our highest calling. Please open your mind to a life-transforming paradigm shift. It may very well require that you open your mind, complete this book (which means to read and actively participate in it), and enjoy the inevitable healing that results in all realms.

How Quantum Physics Shows the Power of Your Mind

At the Rice Diet Program, I usually introduce the subject of quantum physics and its relevance to health by showing the movie *What the Bleep Do We Know!?* and following it with a discussion. The film is an amazing compilation of interviews with the world's top quantum physicists, interwoven with a dramatic thread of "real life" scenes acted by Marlee Matlin, all of which illustrate numerous aspects of quantum physics, such as the law of attraction, the uncertainty principle, and the principle of complementarity. Although the movie is a must-see and impossible to summarize in a few words, I will share some of the pivotal quantum truths it discloses: "Quantum physics is the physics of possibilities. . . . Atoms are not things, they're possibilities. . . . What's happening within us creates what happens outside us. . . . Modern materialism and religion can strip responsibility from the individual; quantum physics can assist one in restoring this responsibility to the individual. . . . Historically, the majority of what people have believed is not true. . . . If you can't control your emotional self, you must be addicted to it. . . . The same receptor sites that attach heroin to our cells attach to emotions as well. . . . Most people don't influence their world much because they don't believe that they can!" Wow! These truths and tantalizing possibilities are truly mind-boggling. Quantum physicist Dr. Fred Alan Wolf ends the show by asking us to think on that for a while. Yeah, right, as if we're capable of deep thought after he and his colleagues have just blown what's left of our minds with a million challenging things to consider. Yet being bombarded and challenged by the fact that most of what we believe is probably not true (and, historically, this has much evidence to support it) jogs our brains and expands our minds to really start reevaluating everything we catch ourselves thinking.

Many people have described how they started to think about this concept: "Well, if my thoughts, feelings, and beliefs do greatly contribute to what happens next in my life, what do I want to start thinking, feeling, and believing that I can do? And if I am really that responsible for everything that I attract and create, how do I begin to forgive myself for past choices and get on with responsibly pursuing what I really want to co-create from this moment on?" This thinking is so radically different from what most Westerners were raised to believe that many Ricers have returned the next day with more questions, such as "How do I begin thinking this way?" and "How will I know if this works?" It is as if their brain freeze had begun to thaw, and they shifted out of autopilot and began to examine their gear-shifting mechanism! Although I have now seen the film dozens of times with the Ricers, who appreciate having a facilitator present for the discussion afterward, the film always reinspires me to reawaken to the abundant power within me and to remember that it is an ongoing choice and opportunity.

At the Rice Diet Program we sleep on it, and usually the next day I lead an experiential from Dr. Fred Alan Wolf's *Dr. Quantum Presents: A User's Guide to Your Universe*. This six-CD set colorfully summarizes the history of quantum physics and laces it with inspiring stories and challenges. His story about the magician's boxes (disc 2, track 4), inspired by William Newcomb, describes the principle of complementarity, which was first proposed by Niels Bohr: "What you get depends upon what you choose." Our thoughts, our intentions, our dreams, our beliefs that we can or cannot do something make all the difference in the world. We have the choice to decide whether we see particles (fixed options) or waves of possibilities (infinite options). Dr. Wolf believes this is how consciousness affects the world, our lives, and our bodies. I play the CD for my group and write this challenging proposal on the board, because that way its unusual premise is often easier for us to see and hear in order to fully grasp.

A wizard or wise man explains that you can choose the right box *or* both boxes. If you choose both box, you are guaranteed that the left box contains $1,000, and it is yours, no questions asked. The right box contains either nothing ($0) or $1,000,000! The wizard says, "I will make you rich if you believe in my power. You must have faith in me and you must have that faith to get the $1,000,000. What you get depends upon what you choose. But if you are greedy you will just get the $1,000." These are paradoxical to your mind only because what you believe: you believe what is "out there" is already "out there" independent of your choice! We have the choice to decide whether we see particles or waves of possibilities. We have the choice to believe we can actualize and co-create the health, dreams, and life we desire, or not!

This experiential is a mind bender because we tend to think our choices in life are either in the left or right box (i.e., either/or options) and that it's not possible for us to positively affect the outcome of our choices. We also tend to think that more is better, so when in doubt, take both. But as Dr. Wolf's story suggests, these belief systems are not necessarily true. The wizard in the story is challenging us to examine whether we can believe that what he said is true—that he has the power to co-create our best outcome—or that we should take what is guaranteed and safe. These questions, like many that quantum physics has posed, invite us to reexamine the way we think and unintentionally limit ourselves and to consider whether our thoughts are co-creating what we want.

This story always leads to interesting aha moments about paradigm shifts, or changes in our unconscious assumptions about how things are, or how our thoughts and choices have influenced various situations in our past. It can help us see whether we have a benevolent or abundant expectation from the Creative Source of the Universe, or instead we come from a scarcity-based belief system—and take what we can get, which is better than nothing. Most of us reading this were raised in an affluent society, yet many of our parents and grandparents survived the Great Depression, World War II, or the Holocaust, so their deep-seated feelings of deprivation, scarcity, and fear that things might very well get worse are understandable, yet are often not that beneficial and applicable to the next generation. It is similar to how our ancestors responded physiologically to a threat by elevating their blood pressure and heart rate to outrun a sabertooth tiger or an invading army. This may have served their escape efforts, yet it doesn't help their descendants' response to a traffic jam many generations later. Our neurological wiring is physiological, as well as highly influenced by our thoughts and beliefs that our forebears and our culture have passed down to us. The more we recognize this and become aware that we are reacting because of old memory wiring, rather than based on something in true, present-moment reality, the more we will experience transformational awakenings to the creative power we hold within us.

Interestingly enough, Eastern thought is filled with the belief that we have power over our destiny through our minds. Recently, in *Train Your Mind Change Your Brain*, Sharon Begley, a *Wall Street Journal* science writer, gave us insight into the late-2004 meetings between leading Western scientists and the Dalai Lama at his home in Dharamsala, India. They answered the question "Is it really possible to change the structure and function of the brain, and thus how we think and feel?" with a resounding yes! Begley goes on to state:

> The discovery that mere thought can alter the very stuff of the brain is another natural point of connection between the science of neuroplasticity and Buddhism. Buddhism has taught for twenty-five hundred years that the mind is an independent force that can be harnessed by will and attention to bring about physical change. "The discovery that thinking

something produces effects just as doing something does is a fascinating consonance with Buddhism," says Francisca Cho [a professor in East Asian Buddhism and culture at Georgetown University]. "Buddhism challenges the traditional belief in an external, objective reality. Instead, it teaches that our reality is created by our own projections; it is thinking that creates the external world beyond us. The neuroscience findings harmonize with this Buddhist teaching."

Buddhist narratives have another consonance with the discoveries of neuroplasticity. They teach us that by detaching ourselves from our thoughts, by observing our thinking dispassionately and with clarity, we have the ability to think thoughts that allow us to overcome afflictions such as being chronically angry. "You can undergo an emotional reeducation," Cho says. "By meditative exertion and other mental exercises, you can actively change your feelings, your attitudes, and your mind-set."

I highly recommend contacting the Jon Kabat-Zinn meditation practice group (see the resources) to find out whether the group has an upcoming session near you.

If you are a religious person, you may think that you would be more comfortable if your thoughts and mind were directed toward God. These meditation techniques are not religious practices. And I am not suggesting that quantum physics and Buddhism or any other meditative approaches are recommended techniques to offer you salvation and the ultimate spiritual experience. I am simply suggesting that they can provide a way for you to nurture mindfulness and a more conscious way of being. (Indeed, chapter 5 will focus on connecting with your spirit and delving into the health advantages of having a relationship with God, a Higher Power, or Universal Truth.) For now, simply recognize here that your mind possesses the ability to harness and co-create the purpose that you believe you are called to fulfill. Given that most of our food consumption and lifestyle choices are not done mindfully, and that the majority of our diseases are the result of our unconsciously choosing disease-promoting lifestyles, it is key that we awaken to the power of our minds to co-create the health that we want. Furthermore, recognizing our power to control our thoughts and thus our feelings and opening to the truth within us all is essential for our long-term success at realizing and sustaining the optimal health and lives we desire.

Until you discover a technique that suits you, simply find a quiet, comfortable place, breathe slowly and deeply for a few breaths, then watch your breath and follow it with your mind's eye as it flows into your toes. Breathe out any tension with your exhalation, as the breath leaves your feet, legs, hips, torso, fingers, arms, shoulders, face, and so on. As you breathe in again, return to any areas where you sense that tension remains. Then simply sit with yourself, enjoying the peace or noticing the thoughts that arise. If you practice this daily, you will not only enjoy physiological improvements (lower blood pressure, heart rate, reduction in platelet stickiness, and so on), you will also experience more moments of mindfulness and peace.

Day 12: *Watch* What the Bleep Do We Know!? *and Listen to* Dr. Quantum Presents: A User's Guide to Your Universe

Enhance your understanding and openness in regard to healing your mind. Watch the film *What the Bleep Do We Know!?* It's available in most video rental stores. Then journalize on what comes up for you. For those of you who haven't bought or found a journal in order to participate in these exercises, at least go get a piece of paper now. It is time to enroll your mind, reconnect with your heart and spirit, and take some action! After you watch this mind-expanding compilation of practical and powerful quantum physics research studies, journalize on what you really want to co-create.

For those who want to venture farther down the rabbit hole, listen to *Dr. Quantum Presents: A User's Guide to Your Universe*; see the resources for ordering information.

The awareness that your mind affects material reality, whether you actualize the results you intend, is hardly a new concept. Neither is it restricted to the level of subatomic particles. It readily translates into helping you achieve what you most desire. This secret to success was brilliantly and practically summarized by Napoleon Hill in 1937 in what became the best-selling success book of all time, *Think and Grow Rich*. The seed for this book was planted by Andrew Carnegie into the brain of Mr. Hill more than a quarter of a century before the book was written. Carnegie provided access for Mr. Hill to interview more than five hundred of the wealthiest and most effective people of that era, including Henry Ford, Teddy Roosevelt, William Wrigley, Wilbur Wright, William Jennings Bryan, Woodrow Wilson, William Howard Taft, Alexander Graham Bell, John D. Rockefeller, F. W. Woolworth, and Thomas A. Edison. Napoleon Hill carefully analyzed their success and summarized his findings of their use of "the secret." Although we all know that education can be important in helping us achieve what we want to create, Hill clearly stated that IQ is not nearly as powerful a determining predictor of success as the implementation of "the secret" is. He shares how Thomas A. Edison, who had only three months of schooling, became the world's leading inventor by intelligently employing "the secret."

While "the secret" is not really a secret, it is not easily obtained in school. It is found as we seek our definite purpose and deepest desire. The word *educate* is derived from the Latin *educo*, which means "to educe, to draw out, to develop from within." A few of the many coaching tips Napoleon Hill shared include developing a definite desire and being ready to receive it, the importance of converting defeat into stepping-stones of opportunity, becoming success conscious (seeking abundance versus scarcity consciousness), maintaining open-mindedness, and determining and documenting your goal with action plans and specific dates. As quantum physics research has repeatedly shown, energetic quantum leaps occur when people think, feel, know it as truth, and act.

The Power of Our Words

In a recent group at the Rice Diet Program, we discussed the healing power of the spoken word and the importance of honesty and integrity imbuing everything that comes from our mouths and enters our ears. I gave a few examples of how often I hear participants come in talking about "my arthritis" or how they have "inherited my heart disease" or that they are overweight "because all the members of my family are just big people." Even those of us who strive to speak only the truth will catch ourselves doing otherwise, but the more we become mindful of what we say and hear, the more intentional we will become about saying what we really mean. Tapping into the truth within us and consistently speaking from this source will release power.

I experienced this firsthand. After at least five years of saying that I knew I was supposed to write a book on the history and efficacy of the Rice Diet, "but I didn't have time," I finally figured out that I was limiting my own power to do so. I had chanted the mantra "but I don't have time" for years, until one day it became very clear to me that by doing so, I was creating a reality that included not having enough time. This particular shift in consciousness occurred during a group experiential, where I stood in front of a large room full of people and stated, "I will sell this book to a major publishing house by July 31."

In less than a month, a front-page *New York Times* business section article titled "Durham, the Weight Loss Capital of the World" focused on the Rice Diet Program and our many successful participants. The very next day, a senior editor from Simon & Schuster called me to see if they could publish my next book. When I said that I wondered how I would sell this by July 31, because I wanted the book in stores by the following January, she explained that I would have to have the entire manuscript completed by July 31—not only sold by then! This successful book was birthed in less than two months, immediately after I quit chanting that I didn't have enough time!

At first, it may sound simple and also crazy that words can actually have so much power, but they do. If you don't yet believe it, over the next month meditate and journalize about what you have thought and felt about what comes out of your mouth, as well as about the conversations around you. Also challenge a friend who is interested in experiencing a shift in his or her life to join you in the exercise of pointing out to each other when you use the following disabling phrases, or "back door open" expressions. A "back door open" response is vague and noncommittal, giving you a way out before you've barely made it through the door. An example of this would be if you asked someone to dinner on a certain date and she said, "I'll try." Would you bet money on the likelihood of her coming? Probably not. In this way, the use of the word "try" undermines a person's intention and becomes almost wishy-washy. The next time you insert the word "try" in relation to a purpose or a goal you would like to achieve, take a moment to reflect on the degree of your commitment: are you only going to try? Or are you going to go for it? The use of disabling words will not help you achieve your goal of healing and develop awareness and integrity with what you say, thus create. Say what you mean; mean what you say. It is okay to change your plans; simply do your best to pursue the completion of your stated intentions.

Getting in touch with what you really want and becoming aware that what you think, speak, and hear can positively and intentionally support your achievement of your goal. Louise Hay's *You Can Heal Your Life* has many pages of positive affirmations that have benefited numerous people as they consciously chose to replace negative sayings or thought patterns with positive, empowering

Words That Disable	Words That Empower
Try	Do (think Yoda from *Star Wars*)
My arthritis	My joints are healing
Suppose to, have to, ought to	Choose to, get to
My bad knee or back	My healing knee or back
I've inherited obesity	A genetic propensity is not as strong a factor as my *dieta*
I don't have enough willpower	I can amaze myself with my focus and follow-through
I hope	I will
Decide	Choose

ones. Practicing these commitments and positively supporting yourself with other introspective practices, such as yoga, journalizing, and playing or listening to music, especially in concert, will ready you for the quantum leap you seek.

Develop Your Positivity

Recently, I had the pleasure of meeting Dr. Barbara Fredrickson. Dr. Fredrickson entered the positivity research arena soon after its inception in the late 1990s, and she addressed certain key points that have helped establish its recent success. Although her mentors were some of the first leaders in the field, she charted a new course by proposing that unlike negative emotions, which narrow people's ideas about possible actions, positive emotions actually do the opposite. She developed the broaden-and-build theory of positive emotions to show that positive emotions open us; they open our hearts and minds, which in turn inspires more receptiveness and creativeness and builds these psychological strengths into habits until we feel a newfound sense of purpose and resiliency within ourselves and in our lives.

It is beyond exciting to observe her ability to design and implement studies that identify which aspects of positivity are most effective and how to translate these into practical suggestions for developing more positivity, health, and love in our lives. All of us probably think that positive feelings are good, but her recent book, *Positivity*, beautifully summarizes what is really so good about feeling good. Her research inspires you to want to cultivate more positive emotions in your life, to enjoy the many proven benefits she cites—from more success in your marriage, a larger salary, and better health to greater longevity (up to ten years longer). Who wouldn't want these fruits?

Although many forms of positivity fill our days, she walks you through the research that specifically addresses the following ten emotions: joy, gratitude, serenity, interest, hope, pride, amusement, inspiration, awe, and love. Her research suggests and has been repeatedly confirmed by others that we would all greatly benefit from a positivity to negativity ratio of 3 to 1. Although 80 percent of people taking the Positivity Self Test that follows (see pages 120–121) score less than this, and average scores are around 2 to 1, she provides plenty of evidence that we are trainable and that by practicing the numerous recommended techniques, we will be able to increase our ratio and thus improve our odds for enjoying optimal health and an upward spiral toward flourishing.

Because emotions arise from how we interpret life events and ideas as they occur, the essence of improving our positivity ratio is becoming more aware of what we think and feel and then take responsibility for choosing to nurture positive thoughts and feelings. In addition, Dr. Fredrickson's book documents research that has shown that people who practiced the positivity techniques were healthier and had fewer sore throats, less nausea, less acne, lower levels of stress-related hormones and higher levels of growth-related and bond-related hormones, higher dopamine and opioids, enhanced immune system functioning, and diminished inflammatory responses to stress. Dr. Fredrickson states that with positivity, "you are literally steeped in a different biochemical stew," so it's little wonder that the health benefits go on and on. Positivity also brings lower blood pressure, less pain, fewer colds, better sleep, and less hypertension, diabetes, and strokes, and did I mention that it increases longevity? Yes, that, too!

Well, how do we get and maintain this positivity? A first step is by taking up meditation, which requires only ten to twenty-five minutes per day. In one of Dr. Fredrickson's experiments, she purposely created anxiety in her subjects by telling them they would be videotaped making a speech, which is a proven way to threaten the majority of people. They were also told that they might be placed in a group that would see a movie and be exempt from making a speech. While they watched the movie and began to think, Yeah, I'm in the movie group, their cardiovascular reactions shifted from panic after experiencing the speech threat to a more relaxed state. This showed that positivity can quell or undo the cardiovascular aftereffects of negativity within seconds to more than a minute. Those who were shown movies evoking serenity or amusement experienced the undoing faster than those who were shown negative or neutral-type movies. When you realize that you are anxious, you can help your heart recover with serenity or amusement-producing media. We all experience stress. It is empowering to know that the stress is not nearly as harmful as your response to it—and you have the choice to exercise your power by choosing relaxing and humorous activities over nail biting and hand wringing!

Although positivity ratios are in part inherited from your family, science has shown that this is only half of the story. The other half depends on a combination of circumstances and how you choose to think and respond. You are never too old to learn; it is your choice to practice meditation, journalize, and be mindful of how you respond to what some people call stress. You can literally train yourself to view this as an opportunity to reframe the way you look at and experience your life.

Although my brother learned the same anger and control-ridden responses that I did as a child, he can make lemons out of lemonade faster than anyone I know. Within twenty-four hours of his lakefront home burning to the ground, he called me and told me what had happened and about everything that was destroyed.

No more than two minutes into the conversation, he got excited and said,

> You know, as awful as this is, few people get to design and build their own dream home, and fewer still get to do it twice. . . . I always wished my kitchen was a few feet wider, and I think I'll change the garage entry so I don't have to walk through the laundry room. You know, it's a shame that new Lexus went up in smoke, too, but I think I'll get the color I really wanted this time!

I'm serious, folks—I'll bet he shifted into the possibilities that this tragedy offered faster than anyone in history ever has! Those who have developed resiliency make use of positivity and openness. This gives them a wide lens, to appreciate the present moment (my brother and his family were all unharmed) and to find the good within the bad (yes, bigger kitchen, better house layout, and newer car in preferred color).

Let's see where we each stand by taking Dr. Fredrickson's Positivity Self Test. This test can be taken here (see below) and hand calculated or taken and tabulated more quickly on her Web site, www.PositivityRatio.com.

I challenge you to take the Positivity Self Test daily for at least one month. Let it give you valuable and concrete evidence, much as your scale does with daily weight checks. I would also recommend taking the test at the same time of day if you can. Although this is less crucial than your timing in weighing yourself, it does help create a habit that can serve you well over the long haul. Dr. Fredrickson's Web site not only scores you automatically, it also tracks your positivity ratio week by week, month by month, and year by year. As with the diet itself, there is nothing like great results to fuel and stoke your ongoing commitment to succeed. You simply need to choose a user name and a password and indicate whether you want to contribute your scores to the growing database maintained by Dr. Fredrickson's research lab. Your first visit will take no more than five minutes and thereafter only a minute to complete. It's like brushing your teeth; simply do it for your health and sparkling smile!

Day 13: Positivity Self Test

How have you felt during the last twenty-four hours? Look back over the previous day and, using the 0–4 scale, indicate the degree that you've experienced each of the following feelings.

0 = not at all
1 = a little bit
2 = moderately
3 = quite a bit
4 = extremely

1. What is the most amused, fun-loving, or silly you felt?
2. What is the most angry, irritated, or annoyed you felt?

3. What is the most ashamed, humiliated, or disgraced you felt?
4. What is the most awe, wonder, or amazement you felt?
5. What is the most contemptuous, scornful, or disdainful you felt?
6. What is the most disgust, distaste, or revulsion you felt?
7. What is the most embarrassed, self-conscious, or blushing you felt?
8. What is the most grateful, appreciative, or thankful you felt?
9. What is the most guilty, repentant, or blameworthy you felt?
10. What is the most hate, distrust, or suspicion you felt?
11. What is the most hopeful, optimistic, or encouraged you felt?
12. What is the most inspired, uplifted, or elevated you felt?
13. What is the most interested, alert, or curious you felt?
14. What is the most joyful, glad, or happy you felt?
15. What is the most love, closeness, or trust you felt?
16. What is the most proud, confident, or self-assured you felt?
17. What is the most sad, down-hearted, or unhappy you felt?
18. What is the most scared, fearful, or afraid you felt?
19. What is the most serene, content, or peaceful you felt?
20. What is the most stressed, nervous, or overwhelmed you felt?

You'll notice that each item within the Positivity Self Test casts a wide net. Each includes a trio of words that are related but are not quite the same. With this strategy, each item captures a set of emotions and all of the feelings share a key resemblance.

If you do not have access to Dr. Fredrickson's Web site, which instantly tabulates your positivity ratio, you can compute your own by following these five simple steps:

1. Go back and circle the ten items that reflect positivity.
2. Go back and underline the ten items that reflect negativity.
3. Count the number of circled positivity items that you scored as 2 or higher.

4. Count the number of underlined negativity items that you scored as 1 or higher.
5. Calculate the ratio by dividing your positivity tally by your negativity tally. If your negativity count is zero for today, consider it instead to be a 1, to sidestep the can't-divide-by-zero problem. The resulting number represents your positivity ratio for today.

As stated earlier, if you scored below 3 to 1 you've got plenty of company—about 80 percent of the population will have this score, but one month of practicing your mindfulness meditation and other recommended offerings in this chapter will improve this. If your ratio is persistently as low as 1 to 1, Dr. Fredrickson suggests that you seek professional assistance. Considering that depression affects one in five people, it would be worth having yourself assessed. She also mentions that the National Institutes of Mental Health has an excellent, user-friendly online brochure currently available at www.nimh.nih.gov/health/publications/depression/nimhdepression.pdf.

Literally hundreds of scientific studies show us that when people change their thinking, they change their emotions as well. So, commit to your meditation practice, and invite all of your senses to the healing party. This is better known as the "so you think, so you will feel, believe, and 'act as if' way of life." Because we basically make up everything we believe, on one level, why not make it up as you want it to be, rather than fearing what you don't want it to be?

Meditation Can Take You There

Another profoundly simple way to develop positivity is through a gently cultivated meditation practice. In the early 1980s, Jon Kabat-Zinn borrowed from the Buddhism meditation tradition to develop a practice he taught to his Boston patients called mindfulness-based stress reduction, or MBSR (see the resources). As he put it, "Mindfulness means paying attention in a particular way, on purpose, in the present moment, and nonjudgmentally."

When you practice this way of being in the moment, it releases you from the tortuous loop that your negative thoughts can often create by igniting negative feelings. Whereas, when you are present with your negative thought and realize that it is a negative thought and that this, too, will pass, you diffuse it and prevent it from hijacking your feelings into an obsessive or depressive emotional feeding frenzy. Scientific research has shown that mindfulness training literally changes your brain. A mindfulness practice alters the basic metabolism in your brain circuits that is known to underlie emotional responses; it reduces activity in circuits linked with negativity, while increasing activity in circuits linked with positivity. It epitomizes empowerment when you realize that by choosing to practice mindfulness meditation, you are creating new neuronal circuitry that will continue to facilitate the changes you desire in your thinking and feeling, which, of course, will influence your actions and affect your results.

If you have never tried to meditate, the following brief description will get you started before you buy other books (found in the resources) that are devoted solely to teaching mindfulness meditation. I must admit that I have taken the MBSR course at least three times and continue to find it an invaluable experience to reinforce and deepen my practice.

At the Rice Diet Program, we teach participants about the many benefits of meditation. It is an effective tool in stress management. It calms our restless minds and allows us to see things more as they really are. The practice often helps us appreciate our bodies more. And ultimately, it brings us to the present moment, the only moment in which we are living, the only moment in which we can be truly aware of our thoughts and feelings. Read through the instructions once on how to practice this meditation, go to a quiet place, and set a timer for how long you desire to practice (so that you won't be distracted by a concern about passing time). My husband, our primary meditation instructor, shares his approach to the practice below.

Day 14: Meditation Practice

The three main formal meditation exercises at the Rice Diet Program are all based on what Thich Nhat Hanh calls conscious breathing. In all of these exercises, you first bring your awareness to your breathing, so that, breathing in, you know that you are breathing in, and breathing out, you know that you are breathing out. It is helpful to identify where in your body you feel your breath most strongly. If you are breathing abdominally (and this is preferred), then you will feel your belly moving out on the inbreath and back in on the outbreath. This happens quite naturally if your abdominal muscles are relaxed: to breathe in, your diaphragm (the muscle separating your chest from your abdomen) contracts, pushing down into your abdominal cavity and causing your lungs to expand and your belly to stick out. On the outbreath, the diaphragm relaxes, moving back up into your chest, allowing your belly to move back in. Or, if you are breathing through your nose (again, the preferred method), you may feel the cool air at your nostrils on the inbreath and the warm air on the outbreath. Or you may feel your chest moving. Whatever you feel strongest helps you keep your awareness on your breathing. Alternatively, you may say "in" on the inbreath and "out" on the outbreath to help you concentrate on your breathing. As you continue to follow your breathing, you will sooner or later find that your mind has wandered off. When you realize that this has happened, notice where you have gone and how you are feeling. You may also note that you are no longer aware of your breathing. Just bring your awareness back to your breathing. Each time your mind wanders off, notice where it has gone and how your body feels and bring your awareness back to your breathing. You can continue for ten, twenty, thirty, or more minutes. It will be helpful, especially in the beginning of your practice, to use CDs to help you to concentrate. We use Thich Nhat Hanh's *Plum Village Meditations* CDs and Jon Kabat-Zinn's *Mindfulness Meditation* practice CDs and tapes, series 1, 2, and 3 for this purpose. (See the resources for more information.)

We also regularly do two guided meditations. The first is a body scan. The body scan is very relaxing and, if done while lying down, will often put you to sleep. The purpose is not to fall asleep but to be aware of your body and how it feels. The fact that we live mainly in our minds is one reason that we take such poor care of our bodies. We often pay attention to our bodies only when there is a problem. We seldom thank our bodies for continuing to perform, despite the abuse that we visit on them. The *Plum Village Meditations* CD contains a guided meditation in which we smile in thanks to various parts of our bodies: "Breathing in, I'm aware of my heart. Breathing out, I smile to my heart." Jon Kabat-Zinn's series 1 CDs contain a body scan in which we bring our awareness to various parts of our bodies and any feelings in those parts. We imagine that we are breathing into and out from each part in turn.

The second guided meditation that we regularly do is a loving-kindness meditation. Loving-kindness is the desire and capacity to bring joy to ourselves and others. You bring your awareness to your breathing and then to your "heart space" in the center of your chest. You then bring up feelings of joy, love, and kindness and send these feelings to five people: yourself, a friend or a mentor, a neutral person (someone you've met or seen but don't really know), a loved one, and a difficult person. You then return to yourself, to one another, if you are in a group, to all people, to animals and plants and the earth and the Universe. The actual feeling may at first be difficult to bring up and even harder to maintain. If you practice visualizing a person or a pet whom you truly adore, it is obviously the best way to establish the knowledge and confidence that you can do this. We use these words to reinforce the feelings: "May I be happy, may I be healthy, may I be peaceful, may I be safe. And may you be happy, may you be healthy, may you be peaceful, may you be safe." If you wish, you can coordinate the phrases to your breathing: one phrase for the inbreath and another for the outbreath.

Balance Your Brain

In 1968, psychobiologist Roger W. Sperry found that the human brain uses two fundamentally different modes of thinking: the left side of the brain is verbal, analytical, and sequential, and the right side is visual, perceptual, and simultaneous. He would later receive a Nobel

Prize for his research on the functions of the human brain's hemispheres. Our culture has grown to believe that the "three Rs" (reading, [w]riting, and [a]rithmetic), essential for training specific, verbal, numerical, and analytical ways of thinking, are somehow more important than the artistic realm of education, which is considered enriching or valuable but not essential. Yet because the right brain's way of responding is to see the whole picture, it is obviously to our benefit to consciously befriend and nurture both sides of the brain. Our encouragement of a right-brain, big-picture perspective is especially beneficial when we explore issues that have emotional and spiritual roots, such as this introspective examination and inner healing journey. In fact, it could be easily argued that most of our personal and societal stress and suffering could be alleviated or healed by more frequent use of our right brain's wide-angle lens, rather than our left brain's analytical and critical perspective, which often limits our options to linear, scarcity-based solutions. Exercising the right brain is empowering and greatly facilitates our inner healing process. Although we cannot neatly divide up the functions of the brain into right and left halves, because individuals and genders differ, the bottom line is that we need to engage both sides of the brain if we are to flourish.

Not only has our society pushed a predominantly left-brain education on us, most of us also have a natural tendency to feel that left-mode thinking is easier. In contrast, the right brain, or R-mode strategy, may at first seem difficult, unfamiliar, and even a little scary. As Dr. Betty Edwards, in *The New Drawing on the Right Side of the Brain*, describes R-mode thinking, it "must be learned in opposition to the 'natural' tendency of the brain to favor L-mode because, in general, language dominates. By learning to control this tendency for specific tasks, one gains access to powerful brain functions often obscured by language." Dr. Edwards has spent years teaching others how to draw from the right side of the brain. The same magical access or shift into right-brain wisdom also occurs in nondominant hand journalizing. While Dr. Edwards's goals are to teach others to draw and to make cognitive shifts to R-mode, the thinking-seeing mode that is specialized for drawing, ours are to express through writing our deep thoughts and feelings about who we are, why we

are here, and what most fuels our passion to create and love ourselves, others, and our earth. In accessing this wisdom and inherent
knowledge, we will co-create our personal healing and that of our
community and environment.

Drawing and journalizing with the nondominant hand are two
of the most powerful ways to connect and realize in a deep way
that this science of the brain is real and is worthy of our further
exploration. I have led nondominant-hand journalizing sessions at
the Rice Diet Program, in which I asked participants to write about
whatever first popped into their minds once they were in a meditative, alpha-wave state. I always remind them that they can trust that
whatever comes up is indeed what they need to journal on; this is
not an exercise on how to squelch undesired thoughts but how to
attend to those that come up.

One example comes to mind of a woman in her forties, who
had no previous memory of sexual abuse. During the introductory
meditation time, a memory of an uncle whom she disliked popped
into her head; the recollection of him troubled her. When she questioned what she should do with that, I asked her whether she would
mind simply writing with her dominant hand: Why are you here
today? Why should I remember you today? Then to place the pen
in her nondominant hand and allow him to answer the questions.
When you take such a stretch, because you aren't your uncle, you
simply relax and imagine him and listen to whether you can sense
what he might say if he were available to answer.

She began to journalize with her nondominant hand, and tears
poured from her eyes. This simple exercise had unlocked the long-
hidden memory (by her left brain, or ego) of sexual abuse by her
uncle. It had remained secured deep within her brain until she was
able to handle the full truth of her past. The exercise with the nondominant hand had freed the right brain to release the buried pain to
her consciousness when she was mature and emotionally ready
to deal with it. I had previously heard that you can be in your forties
before you even remember a childhood trauma as dramatic as sexual
abuse, but I had never seen such a pain release into the light of consciousness through a journalizing exercise. I truly do not think this

would have happened without the nondominant hand aspect being exercised, but we will never know. It was the most amazing example I can recall of how the conscious mind, which is largely left-brain driven, can seek more brain assistance, literally by inviting the right brain to participate, to expand and open, and allow us depths of healing that were not available to our analytical, critical, everyday way of thinking. Obviously, when this Ricer gained full knowledge of her painful past, of her early need to eat for comfort, of her need to bury the dirty family secret and protect herself by hiding under layers of unhealthy fat, she was more able to lose weight and finally keep it off! Without gaining access to this right-brain knowledge of her past, thus of herself, she would not even be aware of the years of deep, destructive thoughts she had of herself: that she was not worthy, that she was a victim and somehow deserved to be one. Knowledge is indeed power, and often we do not have full access to our own truths unless we regularly engage the right brain and know ourselves at deeper levels, literally know our roots so that we can accept the healing that is available for us to receive.

In all of my expressive writing and journalizing classes, I gently caution participants of the profundity of this practice. It can often unleash more issues than you expected, but with access to great psychiatrists and psychotherapists, we have never had a Ricer regret this cathartic exploration. You may want to ask your doctor or other respected health practitioner if he or she can recommend a psychotherapist in case you release more pain than you care to process alone.

Day 15: Nondominant Hand Journalizing

Write the following question with your dominant hand: "What have I been feeding, or hungry for, this past year while gaining fifty pounds?" Or write another probing question that is true for you and relevant to your goal, such as "How is it serving me to stay in this dead-end job or relationship, and what do I fear about choosing to change it?"

Then put the pen in your nondominant hand and write the answer. Allow yourself to answer from your heart, accessing the right-brain wisdom; it is often helpful to remind yourself that your six-year-old self can speak and be heard. Your writing will look like a first grader's, and often your answers are found during the memories of these younger years. So let your inner child have a word with you. My first attempt with nondominant hand journalizing produced: "This really feels stupid. I bet this is a waste of time!" So don't worry if your more practiced, critical left brain does not want to relinquish its command of the situation; just stick with it, breathe deeply for a few breaths, and ask your inner child what his or her thoughts are. Mentally remind your right brain that it is okay to come out and play. It is natural and quite common for this to take a while, so allow yourself at least fifteen minutes with this experience, for a few days in a row. Most participants who give it a fair effort are amazed at what comes out!

You Can Do It: Making a Paradigm Shift

Most overweight people I meet quickly explain to me that they "just like food" or that they "come from a large family" or "everyone in my family is big," or "I really don't eat as much as a lot of thin people I know; I can look at food and gain weight." Although I believe that much of this information has some degree of truth in it, it largely evades the important, empowering truth—which would include what their minds have not revealed to them or what they do not care to admit out loud. Because our egos function to secure our need for love, acceptance, security, and approval, we tend to communicate what we think will make us look good or right, or we say whatever we think will be perceived as funny or intelligent. This ego-driven response is not something people are necessarily aware of, it is so deeply ingrained in us—we simply do it out of habit, because we've been working from this survival platform our entire lives. *Webster's* defines *ego*, in psychoanalytic terms, as "the part of the psyche which experiences the external world through the senses, organizes the thought processes rationally, and governs action; it mediates between the impulses of the id (our reservoir of instinctual drives and the source of psychic energy, dominated by the pleasure principle), the demands of the environment, and the standards of the superego (which enforces moral responses)."

Although our culture's ego-dominated approach to thinking and reacting has gotten us this far, we do have a choice to awaken to the deeper truth of why we do what we do and why we habitually do what we don't want to do and to change our thinking to co-create what we really want to do with our lives. A long and tiring battle with overeating or, frankly, any painful condition that we exhaust ourselves with fighting can pivot us into a new realm of thinking. Many people have described to me the moment when they realized that they would do anything rather than continue on their ineffective path of hopelessness or desperation, and when they relinquished the illusion that they were actually in control or "right" about whatever. It was only then that they awakened to their minds' role in contributing to it, as well as their power to change their minds and their future prognoses. This is often described as a paradigm shift, the moment when we first realize we can choose to perceive things differently and then almost instantly and effortlessly do so.

One of the most motivating participants whom we've had the pleasure of pursuing health with is Jan, who is now practically everyone's coach. Jan, like many Ricers, had a life filled with professional accomplishments. She conducted chemistry research and lectured in German for Swiss agricultural and chemical companies, then excelled in selling residential and commercial real estate. But as many of you know, being brilliant and competent doesn't always mean that you remember to prioritize a healthy lifestyle. The excessive hours she devoted to her real estate work, along with her new fast-food habits, led to Jan's overweight status in her forties. In 2002, when she was sixty-two, Jan walked into the Rice Diet Program weighing 216 pounds. She had tried almost every diet in the country and was desperately seeking something that would help her lose her excess weight and finally keep it off. But that was before her cancer. Much to her surprise, Jan was diagnosed with breast cancer only two days into her stay. "I remember going to Dr. Rosati and telling him that I had to drop out," reflects

Jan. "He told me that I wasn't going anywhere … that I was going to stay on the program and get my body healthy before I went through treatment; that is exactly what I did. Before I knew it, the caring staff at the Rice Diet Program had connected me to the best physicians and health-care team at Duke. I received excellent care, and they had *just* met me two days before."

When Jan started radiation therapy, she was walking the Duke Trail (that's 3.2 miles of steep incline and decline) daily. Her oncologist warned her that she might feel lethargic and would probably have to cut back on her exercise. Without a moment of hesitation, Jan looked him square in the face and said, "You wanna bet?" By the end of her treatment, Jan had walked the Duke Trail every single day. Jan later celebrated five years of being cancer-free by hiking to the Mt. Everest base camp (up 17,600 feet).

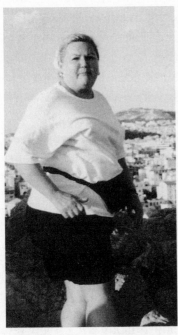

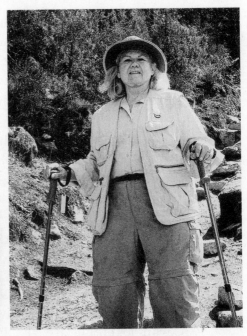

Jan before starting the Rice Diet Program.

Jan afterward, during a trek on Mount Everest.

To get ready for the climb, Jan worked hard with her personal trainer, Greg McElveen, at Duke's Sports Performance Lab.

"I eat more at night when I'm home by myself," says Jan. "When I have someone to talk to who has similar issues as me, I don't feel so alone." Jan says that she has learned a lot from the nutrition classes at the Rice Diet and really likes the psychological support classes that teach her craving management and coping skills.

When asked what keeps her going, Jan says that her biggest motivation is health. "I don't want to be in a wheelchair or nursing home like my mother was," confesses Jan. "I know that if I stay focused, I'll stay healthy. Cancer taught me a lot: that the healing process is powerful and real. It also taught me to appreciate life more and about the importance of living every day like it really matters. Of course, it helped me conquer cancer to have an optimistic and hard-driving approach. I prefer to say that I have conquered it, not just survived it; this says to me that it's gone. I have conquered it and it's over. And I can spend my time and mental energy thinking about trekking the mountains I have yet to climb. I relate more to the verb *conquering*, which is the word that mountain climbers use when they describe a summit that they have reached. I believe if I keep my focus on the next elevation or peak I want to reach, I will be going in that direction, not only with my feet but with my life and health."

Check out Jan's before and after photos (on the previous page), which say more than words can about creating paradigm shifts, opening to new possibilities, and conquering the mountains of our choice.

"Shift Happens" with All of Our Senses

One of our star Ricers, Jean, shared with us that an addiction program had taught her how helpful a craving-management kit could be in inspiring a shift in her obsessive thoughts to overeat. She engaged us with her enthusiasm about how quickly and effectively the kit's contents could inspire her shift from obsessive thoughts to overeat to thoughts of pleasant past memories or fantasies yet to be. This was easy to believe, given our knowledge of how our olfactory response is the fastest sense to be received and processed by the brain. Smells, such as lavender or rose, are processed by the amygdala, a small part of the old brain, which processes significantly faster than our cortex, the rationalizing front part of the brain, can physically react. So keeping a Paradigm Shift Happens Kit handy and easily accessible can quickly help us change gears from obsessing about a second trip to the refrigerator to taking a walk to pursue more enticing smells! Create your own kit and include smells that may save you from yourself; then invite all of your senses to experience healthier possibilities.

Day 16: The Paradigm Shift Happens Kit

At the Rice Diet Program, we have been impressed with the results Ricers have described after creating their own Paradigm Shift Happens Kits. You can create your own unique kit by choosing a small plastic container and filling it with a variety of treasures that will assist you in shifting all of your senses to pleasurable memories or times. You may wish to include a small picture of your dream place to go to in your mind (you can find a photo the size of your container and glue it within the top or roll or fold it to fit inside) and a scent or a fragrance you like. Some people like essential oils of lavender, lemon, or mint, which can instantaneously shift their focus from a food craving to the gardens of their Irish relatives in County Cork or their last tropical vacation. Although certain individuals would find that a quick sniff of a cinnamon stick can immediately take them back to their grandmother's Christmas gatherings of a half century ago, others would let the cinnamon stick catapult them into the nearest Cinnabon store! So be forewarned, this is a very personal exercise that needs your careful attention as to the selection of these key aromatic ingredients. Stimulate your other senses with tactile and auditory reminders. Include a gratitude rock that can inspire your recollection and appreciation for your nature walks, and store your mp3 player loaded with your latest uplifting songs to help shift you to other activities that you enjoy other than eating. Although this is an evolving project for us at the Rice Diet Store, we now sell the basic kits complete with a balloon to remind you to breathe and have more fun!

5

Connecting with Your Spirit

A major need of our being is to know ourselves, to feel the love and acceptance that occur when we are truly known by ourselves, by God, and by our community. The need to be known is ingrained in us. From games like peekaboo to hide and seek, to our meditation and journalizing disciplines, we seek to know ourselves more deeply and clearly so that we can feel more at ease, be more engaged in our lives, and love more fully. This quest for self-knowledge is a deep need and hunger within us all, and if we don't feed it, we often binge on other substitutes in an attempt to sate the need. When we heal our bodies with good food, heal our hearts by letting go of unnecessary negative emotions, and heal our minds by choosing to think positively, all of these acts give us a greater sense of self-knowledge and ultimately truth, which comes by way of the spirit.

What Ricers come to know and what I hope you are beginning to feel and discover in the pages of this book is that the primary, essential, and supreme way that we understand ourselves and thereby reach true healing is through our spiritual source. Spirituality is the seeking of the sacred, the divine essence of who we are. So whether or not you believe in God and are devoted to a particular religion, all of us possess within ourselves a spirit, an essence that connects us to one another, to the planet, and to the Creative energy that exists throughout the Universe.

From my decades of facilitating and participating in soul-baring groups, it is my experience that if we do not receive a big healthy dose of this love, appreciation, and encouragement to truly be ourselves at a young age, our sense of feeling wounded can run deep. It seems that our health and our ability to flourish and actualize our purpose largely depend on our desire to be healed and our willingness to seek and be open to the loving Creative Force within, the revelation or knowledge of our true identity. By desiring to be healed and being open to this source of love within, we can increasingly walk in our true purpose and consciously and habitually choose to love ourselves and others.

From the latest quantum physics findings to the greatest and most ancient spiritual truths and religious traditions, we are repeatedly given the same answers: that love and unity, the connection with God, ourselves, and others—in fact, with everything—give our lives value and a true sense of purpose and meaning. This connection with love and God also literally heals beyond measure.

Dr. Larry Dossey, in his wonderful books *Healing Words*, *Reinventing Medicine*, and *Healing beyond the Body*, has beautifully described how we have viewed and practiced healing and has identified three eras of medicine. Era I, which began in the middle of the nineteenth century, is based on concepts drawn from the classical, mechanical, Newtonian concept of the Universe and is still the predominant model practiced by Western medicine today. Era II, which began in the middle of the twentieth century, began to realize that thoughts, emotions, attitudes, and beliefs influence our health and healing; it became known as mind-body medicine. Dr. Dossey described how Era III, unlike the first two eras, has been able to scientifically prove that our thoughts, intentions, and prayers affect others, at any distance measured, whether or not the receiver is conscious of the mental and spiritual effort that is being expended. Dr. Dossey's *Healing Words* beautifully summarized the wealth of research on a wide range of plants and animals and showed that positive intentions and prayers inspire incredibly significant improvements in healing. He also reported on Dr. Randolph Byrd's research that revealed the strong influence of distant prayer on the recovery of heart patients in a coronary care unit. It, like numerous studies since, showed that prayer works, whether or not the subjects receiving the prayer know that they are being prayed for. This Era III research has been growing quickly for the last couple of decades and has produced the distance healing evidence, now referred to as nonlocal medicine. All of these eras have gifts to offer us on our healing journeys. Let's take a look at a well-documented research effort that exemplifies the potential for nonlocal healing.

One such type of nonlocal healing has been studied in regard to Transcendental Meditation (TM). Research has now repeatedly shown how TM practice and the coherence-creating group response this produces can dramatically reduce violent crime in a community. Four thousand participants in the TM and TM-Sidhi programs of Maharishi Mahesh Yogi assembled in Washington, D.C., from June 7 to July 30, 1993. Consistent with previous research findings, levels of homicides, rapes, and assaults (HRA crimes) dropped 23.3 percent during this time period!

Furthermore, calculation of the steady state gain based on the time series model predicted that a permanent group of four thousand coherence-creating experts in D.C. would have a long-term effect of reducing HRA crimes by 48 percent! Given the high crime history of this and many other U.S. cities, meditation seems to be a much more cost-effective solution than the billions of dollars spent on anticrime measures (such as longer prison sentences and more police), whose effectiveness is far from proven. This is a great example of how attending to the root of our problems through a spiritually inspired approach, rather than chasing the tail of our problems via physical and superficial means, creates true healing, with more evolved, sustainable, and cost-effective results.

Faith Heals

Most of us know by now that our minds and emotions are intimately involved with our physical beings, yet some people still consider it a leap to believe that the spiritual self or essence can significantly influence our health, our well-being, and the health and well-being of others.

Dr. Harold Koenig, one of the world's most respected researchers on the health benefits of practicing a spiritual discipline, knows this scientific literature better than anyone I'm acquainted with. In addition to writing many wonderful books on this subject, he also finds time to occasionally inspire Ricers with practical summaries of the numerous advantages of having a religious and spiritual practice. He is the founder and codirector of the Center for Spirituality, Theology, and Health at Duke University (which conducts interdisciplinary research, scholarship, and education on spirituality, theology, and health and explores the role of faith communities in forming the health of the broader community). Finally, he is a Duke University psychiatrist in gerontology, and his research participants are primarily Christian, Jewish, and Buddhist. So, regardless of your spiritual or religious orientation, his words shed light on the research, as well as on its practical applications. As at the Rice Diet Program, Dr. Koenig graciously shares here from his wealth of professional knowledge and personal wisdom.

We know that the mind and emotions are intricately connected with the natural physiological systems in the body that allow it to heal. Negative emotions such as anxiety, fear, depression, hopelessness, anger, resentment, or even simply boredom, can interfere with the normal operations of the immune, hormonal, and cardiovascular systems.

Religious faith, belief in a God who cares and who loves us, and who has a purpose for every person—no matter what their situation in life or their physical or mental health—helps many people to cope with difficult circumstances that often cause the negative emotions described above. Because of this powerful role that religion serves in helping people to cope, and because of its influences on daily decisions that affect health, faith has the potential to dramatically influence the development of disease, physiological responses to illness, and rates of healing.

Indeed, systematic research has demonstrated exactly this. First, persons who are more religiously involved experience lower rates of depression and recover more quickly from depression. This is especially true for those experiencing serious health problems. In fact, the magnitude of the correlation between religiousness and depression is directly proportional to how much stress or illness the person is currently facing. The more stress, the stronger the inverse correlation between religion and depression. Because religion is such a powerful coping behavior, research can best demonstrate its effects in situations where people have a lot to cope with.

Second, many studies now demonstrate that religious involvement is related to better immune function, lower blood pressure, greater longevity, better cognitive functioning, and slower progression of disability as persons age. This is all very consistent, since we know that depression, anxiety, and other negative emotions are all related to poorer immune function, higher blood pressure, greater risk of heart disease, worse cognitive functioning, greater problems with physical functioning, and shortened longevity. Likewise, religious persons recover more quickly from surgery and have fewer surgical complications. All of this research suggests that religious involvement can affect physical health and healing rates through mechanisms that can be studied scientifically and documented.

Thus, through its effects on helping people to cope with stress, religion can facilitate the healing process or prevent some diseases entirely, and the scientific research to back this up is growing and growing and growing.

If you are by now questioning whether you have a spiritual or religious practice sufficient to inspire your health, much less reduce the crime rate of a major city, or whether this chapter is possibly outside of your comfort zone, let's remember that you can gain access to this same healing power of the spirit without committing to a religion. We are all human beings and have a spiritual nature, with the word *spiritual* defined (by *Webster's*) as "of the spirit or soul" and *soul* defined as "the spiritual, moral or emotional nature . . . credited with the functions of thinking and willing."

In this way, we all possess a spiritual nature. Some choose to exercise their spirit or faith through a religious practice, and others connect with their fellow human beings, the Universe, animals, or nature as a way to explore and express their spiritual core. For the remainder of this book, I invite you to meditate on the unconditional love that we all desire and have never completely received from another human being. Simply be open-minded and open-hearted to the possibility that the unconditional love and acceptance you desire can come from the Creator of the Universe and that this loving, connecting force is within you. Suspend for this time any agenda or habituated practice of judgment about whether you agree or disagree with what we call this Creative Force or Higher Power. Simply be open to the possibility that you can be fully known, loved, and accepted for who you are and can enjoy the health benefits of doing so!

Whether you can really hear and digest this important truth that pervades the latest research in quantum physics, in positivity psychology, or from HeartMath investigators, or perhaps you've discovered it by exploring your own inner sanctuary and/or taking a journey within your religious discipline of choice, the message is consistent everywhere: Become aware of what you *think, feel*, and *believe*, and thus *do* (in other words, your truth), because it matters. We are co-creators with the Creator of the Universe, so we might as well remain mindful of this wonderful gift and use this power wisely.

Journalize: Tap into Your Spirit

I invite you to take this opportunity to explore whatever feelings have come up for you. Many people struggle with delineating the difference between spirituality and religiosity. This is often due to their distress and guilt about their religion's history, the pain they experienced as a result of the behavior of their early spiritual or religious teachers, or childhood conflicts with their parents' religious beliefs and practices and the memories they have unconsciously chosen to retain from these. If you have a strong emotional response to this topic, it is a great opportunity for you to heal in this area. Maintaining walls around your heart harms you more than you know. If my simple introduction of the subject of spirituality and religion triggers in you a physical sensation of resistance, I'll ask you at this time to examine the source of this pain or fear and open yourself to heal it at the root.

Day 17: *Nondominant Hand Journalizing on Your Spiritual Health and/or Your Religious Discipline*

Create a quiet space with approximately twenty minutes of uninterrupted time to journalize your thoughts and feelings about your spiritual health and religious practice. Place the pen in your dominant hand and write a spiritually directed question, such as "How do I feel spiritually at this time—grounded and peaceful with my relationship with the Divine, or disconnected, angry, or confused?" or "If I could speak with the Creator, would I care to address some unresolved issues or have a few questions answered?"

Then, switch the pen to your nondominant hand and answer from your heart, permitting yourself to give voice to the six-year-old within and the freedom to write whatever first comes to your mind—without analyzing, critiquing, or judging the content. Simply answer from your heart. Remember that freely writing whatever comes up for you, without censoring or correcting your grammar, is the way to stimulate your right-brain wisdom, a wellspring of intuitive, creative insight. Remind yourself to trust and receive this insight as if you were a child. Don't construct a sophisticated theological monologue, but allow the Divine to speak through the vulnerability of your nondominant hand.

As you partake in this experiential, open yourself up to a paradigm shift. You then may want to give some spiritual depth to your Paradigm Shift Happens Kit by adding a smell (incense), a song (gospel, Gregorian chants, or other inspiring music on your mp3 player), a visual reminder of your faith (a picture of your spiritual mentor or recent pilgrimage), or a tactile stimulus (holy water or a physical reminder of a profound epiphany) to assist you on your spiritual journey.

Centering Prayer, a Seduction into Holy Silence

Some readers who don't already have an established spiritual or religious practice may wonder how they can further nurture their spiritual health. You may have begun to do the meditation practice described in the last chapter, and now you want to try the centering prayer practice when you find that it resonates with your religious roots.

Although many Christians and non-Christians who became disillusioned with their lack of spiritual experience in their church, synagogue, or mosque have sought Eastern meditation methods, others have discovered the contemplative prayer tradition of the Christian church, which was the norm during the first sixteen centuries after the death of Christ. In the 1500s, contemplative prayer fell out of favor, but it experienced a resurrection in the 1970s and 1980s, inspired by Pope Paul VI's encouragement for its renewal and wonderful writings by Thomas Keating and Morton Kelsey, among others. In Thomas Keating's book *Open Mind Open Heart: The Contemplative Dimension of the Gospel*, he describes how spiritual disciplines, both East and West, are based on the hypothesis that there is something that we can do to enter this journey to Divine union once we have realized that such a possibility exists. He explains that centering prayer is a discipline designed to make the ancient Christian tradition of contemplative prayer more user-friendly to today's average seeker. He describes how centering prayer helps us withdraw our attention from the daily chaos of thoughts, which we tend to identify ourselves with, to focus on a deeper part of ourselves, opening ourselves to the spiritual level of our being. Beneath the incessant flow of debris on the surface of our thoughts is an inner stream of consciousness, which he calls "our participation in God's being."

In a very reader-friendly way, he invites us to take the time to develop our awareness of this level, the level of our being that makes us most human and who we are intended to be. So, in addition to revitalizing ourselves with healthy food, daily exercise, and mental and emotional journalizing and processing techniques, we are also strengthened and healed by these moments of holy silence that can bring us into a deeper renewal.

Visualizing a busy, trash-strewn stream with debris swirling on top, versus the more valuable stillness in the stream's depths, reminded me of other similar parallels. Fast food, convenient junk food, and conventionally farmed food in general are chaotically clustered, unnaturally accessible, and seemingly quickly and readily available, but in actuality, the healthiest sustenance is that which is carefully farmed and patiently cultivated. It is all the same whether we are healing the various aspects of our being or of our world. In both farming our food and cultivating our empowering thoughts, feelings, and faith, we must heal deeply to attain the significant changes and sustainable results we desire.

Day 18: How to Do the Centering Prayer

Thomas Keating's method for teaching centering prayer is simplified as follows:

1. Secure a comfortable position for your body, preferably in a quiet location, and set a gentle wake-up alarm for twenty to thirty minutes.
2. Close your eyes, and choose a sacred word that expresses your intention to open and surrender to God. Any simple one- to two-syllable word that you feel comfortable with is fine.
3. Become aware of this word, and repeat it in your mind whenever you recognize any other thoughts arising. You do not need to move your lips.

The suppression of thoughts is not the goal, nor is the sacred word a directional sign. Keating stated that the sacred word "only directs your intention toward God and thus fosters a favorable atmosphere for the development of the deeper awareness to which your spiritual nature is attracted. Centering prayer is not a way of turning on the presence of God. Rather, it is a way of saying, *Here I am*. The next step is up to God. It is a way of putting yourself at God's disposal; it is He who determines the consequences."

After your twenty- to thirty-minute centering prayer time, you may want to converse with God, but give yourself a few minutes in this delicious place before opening your eyes to the world as you knew it. As with all of the practices introduced in this book, you need to give it a one-month trial. It's recommended that you do this twice a day. For some people, it is a challenge to not do anything for twenty minutes straight, but assure yourself that if you are seriously making yourself totally available for your Creator, twice a day, you will feel a growth spurt of faith. Your faith will begin to flourish in unexpected ways. You may find your awareness of God's presence arising within you during ordinary activities, which you had previously not considered to be spiritual experiences.

The quality of your spiritual life will develop and will allow you to pick up vibrations from a world that you did not previously perceive or know was available to you. As you become a willing receptor, these heavenly transmissions, which were always present, will become available for you to receive.

Seeking Spirituality Everywhere

There are virtually endless avenues to strengthen and enrich your spirituality and faith. In addition to organized religious traditions and communities, every moment of life can be viewed as an opportunity for spiritual expansion, a time to nurture the love and unity that are within us and that surround us, even when they are not obvious or apparent. My ongoing prayers and conscious intentions include my desire to attract and meet other spiritually thirsty and enthusiastic friends and for me to recognize such connections between people and events as God-inspired opportunities, rather than hurrying past them or discounting them as coincidences. For instance, I believe that if I had not sought God's direction for this book's birth so tenaciously, I may very well have overlooked these opportunities as the miracles that I believe they are. The following spiritually inspired experiences illustrate how when we pursue (pray, journal, and share with trusted others) our desires, seek God's way of manifesting them, and act as if we are part of our desires' co-creation by moving toward what draws our mind, heart, and spirit, our visions manifest.

Although such holy happenings occur far more frequently than we realize, I am aware of many experiences of feeling God's purpose and plan and riding the wave of a Creative Force greater than myself that occurred during the birthing of this book. In one period of enthusiasm about how this book was evolving, I visited my dear friend and University of North Carolina roommate who lives in Asheville, North Carolina. She was very excited for me to meet her friend, who had sung "How Can I Keep from Singing?" at her son's funeral. Later that afternoon, he sang it to me outside on a sidewalk near an art fair. It moved me to tears, a feeling that came from a very deep place within me. I was overwhelmed with a profound experience of the Spirit; I felt overcome by unconditional love for my friend and her friend, who not only sang the deepest Irish hymn you could imagine but also transported me through his voice to the funeral that I could not attend. The unconditional love of that song, from that man, in that moment, let me transcend time, space, and the emotional extremes of a mother's greatest fear of losing her only son, while experiencing God's greatest love—the unconditional love that truly heals everything in the instant it is realized. It was one of those "wow" experiences.

Within a few hours, my dear friend took me to meet Wendy Whitson, her favorite Asheville artist, who, soon after her son's death, had painted and delivered to her an impressionistic painting of a forest filled with trees. Her painting, like the others we marveled at in the studio, not only had exquisite beauty, color, and proportion, but on closer inspection I was awed by the depth of the tree trunks, which were covered and textured with glued-on strips of sheet music, and topped with mica flecks she had collected by hand in the nearby Blue Ridge Mountains. The trees bespoke life, life with depth, laced with song, substance, and beauty beyond words. Now, as if this was not enough mind-, heart-, and spirit-expanding joy for one day, I had the pleasure of discovering who Wendy Whitson really is and where she came from. Fortunately, she agreed to share how she used her near-death experience to catapult her into the life she really wanted to live. Her story illustrates how an artist who didn't think she was good enough to paint professionally went from framing other people's art to creating masterpieces.

The last really bad "episode" was seven years ago. Wow. Not breathing. When I describe an asthma attack, I tell people: breathe in deeply and hold it. Now breathe in again while you're still holding the first breath. You see, there's no room for air. It is the most terrifying feeling.

I had been a pretty creative child and graduated from East Carolina with a degree in art. After college, I had a number of interesting jobs—landscaping, photography and graphic design. I moved from Greenville to Chapel Hill, to Atlanta, where I resided when my health downturn began.

I was thirty-five. I'd always been extremely healthy and taken good care of myself by eating right and exercising. Out of the blue, I came down with a sinus infection, and before long, I had full-blown asthma. Within a few months I was having severe attacks, and within a year I had my first "near death" experience. I had a battery of doctors behind me, all scratching their heads. But they were also reading, researching, trying to get to the bottom of why it was such a severe case. I saw pulmonologists, allergists, ENTs, endocrinologists, and even an oncologist who did a bone marrow biopsy. There were hospitalizations for tests and numerous ones for respiratory failure.

I was off and on at my job for about five years before I went on disability, which I did not want to do. I really loved my job and the people I worked with—a large architectural firm, the corporate office. At the same time, I'd taken a weekend trip to Asheville, North Carolina, which happened to coincide with a Studio Stroll in the River Arts District. I went into studio after studio and thought, Maybe I can paint again one day. A seed had been planted. Afterward, my marketing materials, presentations, *everything*, began to take on a new look—lots of layers, very complex. Everyone loved them. All I could dream about was painting again.

Meanwhile, I was having extremely severe attacks. They came on very quickly—within minutes of the onset of an attack, I would need to be intubated. I had one doctor tell me when I woke up in the ICU, "Wendy, we caught you by your heels on your way out the door." This scenario happened multiple times over seven years. By then, I was living on steroids and about fifteen other medications, was on disability full time, so just stayed at home, doing breathing treatments. My husband at the time wondered if I would live through the day—every day.

Through it all, I kept thinking, I'm not *supposed* to be this sick. On the other hand, on awakening in the ICU due to respiratory failure, I'd wonder, God, why am I still here?

And I have to tell you—dying is not so bad. In the blink of an eye, I went from exquisite pain to exquisite freedom. The moments before, I was working hard to breathe, hanging on to life. The will to survive is *strong*. But the instant I let go or was forced to let go, an amazing thing happened. I was completely immersed in the most beautiful feeling I have ever felt. *Love!* Times one million! It was everywhere—and pulling me toward more love. I absolutely wanted to keep going.

This is what I experienced every single time I had respiratory failure. Then I would wake up, always tethered to a gurney in the ICU, breathing apparatus in place.

More years went by, things changed. Namely, I remarried and moved to Asheville, North Carolina. Several years ago, I decided to try my hand at painting again, after a twenty-year hiatus. The urge to try was overpowering compared to the fear of not trying. I *had* to know. A friend told me about an available space. As I drove up to Warehouse Studios, déjà vu hit me hard. Could this be the very same building I'd strolled through so many years ago? Yes—it was!

I stepped into my future work space and felt like I'd come home. I decided to rent the studio for one year and see if I could "get it back." For the entire year, I showed up every day and worked, not liking anything I painted. For the whole year I kept at it, and toward the end of my deadline, I truly loved a painting. One. But that's all it took!

I am now a full-time landscape painter. Living in the Blue Ridge Mountains is certainly very inspiring. But so is living. Every day is a gift. My paintings contain a certain amount of structure, which I like to think of as God's Master Plan. An underlying random grid that represents the organization we find in nature and manifests itself as trees in the forest, stems of flowers, reflections, or, sometimes, as itself. My work varies from impressionistic to abstract and, though described as

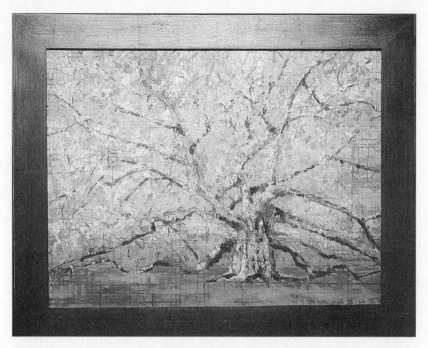

The Angel Oak *by Wendy Whitson is richly textured with strips of actual sheet music, which is glued and painted and then topped with flecks of mica. It is built on top of latticelike lines that Wendy describes as being "anchored on God's grid."*

calm, is also filled with energy. It has been an amazing journey and feels like perhaps this is the reason I'm still breathing.

It was obvious that Wendy's painting and story were given to me for this book—for me to give to you. When Chris and I walked out of Wendy's studio, our minds were both blown at how God had brought me an amazing song, an artist resurrection story, and how it was all so reflective of how we can co-create with the Divine. My friend turned to me with a straight face and simply said, "Kitty, is this the way your life is?" I started to laugh hysterically before admitting, "Well, this would be a very good day!"

The Healing Power of Poetry

From the earliest chants sung by primitive people around tribal fires to the mythological tales of Oceanus, who told Prometheus,

"Words are the physician of the mind diseased," the use of poetry is an ageless approach to healing. When the use of poetry therapy became popular again in the 1960s and 1970s, it was commonly tagged as "bibliotherapy," meaning "the use of literature to serve or help." In one of Freud's more humble moments, he said, "Not I, but the poet discovered the unconscious." Poet and therapist Dr. Perie Longo's succinct summary of poetry therapy stimulated my appreciation for the ancient technique of using rhythmic words to heal.

Dr. Longo clearly sets the foundation for us to take in the historical depth and the interconnected nature of poetry and healing: "The focus of poetry for healing is self-expression and growth of the individual, whereas the focus of poetry as art is the poem itself. But both use the same tools and techniques; language, rhythm, metaphor, sound, and image, to name a few. In the end, the result is often the same. The word *therapy*, after all, comes from the Greek word *therapeia*, meaning 'to nurse or cure through dance, song, poem and drama, that is the expressive arts.' The Greeks have told us that Asclepius, the god of healing, was the son of Apollo, god of poetry, medicine, and the arts historically entwined."

Poetry, possibly more than any genre, connects us with our Creator or the indefinable creative place within us. It comes from a depth that we all have the freedom to tap into, even those who don't consider themselves artistically endowed. Over the years, we have had numerous poets in residence who assisted Ricers who had initially resisted writing poetry. These Ricers were then amazed at the depths they soon divulged and the joy they felt in doing so. Writing and reading poetry of our own or with people we feel connected to can release and satisfy our souls. Dr. Longo adds, "A poem has much to teach us about ourselves and the world, as form and sound give rise to silence. One of the benefits of poetry reading and writing is not only does it help define the 'I,' but strengthens it. This is necessary if we are to be a part of the world. The process attaches us to the greater part of ourselves, to all that is whole and good and beautiful. And when we feel ourselves as not alone in the world, but a part of and integrated with all that exists, self-esteem grows."

World-renowned philosophers, hypnotherapists, brain scientists, and our own endocrinologist and poet in residence, Dr. Frank Neelon, are well aware of the power of the spoken word to inspire change. Learning to do what we really want to do but are not yet doing is key to much health and happiness. People do change. Dr. Neelon beautifully summarizes why we offer poetry at the Rice Diet Program:

People often ask why we use poetry at the Rice House. Why not just stick to "science"? they ask, as though information alone will get us on the right track. My position is that lack of information is not the problem. For example, if I asked each Rice Diet participant to write down the ten things that he or she needs to do to get and to stay healthy, every one of them would get the answers right. But life is not a quiz; rather, it is a struggle between knowing what to do and doing it.

That, I think, is where poetry comes in. Look at poetry as a form of heightened and concentrated speech, speech where every word, every pause, every syllable has meaning. This formulation implies that poems should be heard, not read (and further, that the poems should be recited, not simply read aloud). This formulation allows poetic words to stick in the soul, to become one with the hearer, to stay with the receiver long after the transmitter is silent. The Velcrolike stickiness of good poems puts them in the same class as the therapeutic trance messages delivered by the famous hypnotherapist Milton Erickson, who said, "My voice will go with you." Poems go with you, too.

The cortex (the outer, "thinking" layer) of the human brain comprises two nearly identical halves, only one of which (almost always the left hemisphere) harbors the ability to speak. We know from the elegant observations of Roger W. Sperry and Michael S. Gazzaniga that the right (silent or mute) half of the brain can communicate with the left, both directly (that is, information delivered to the right brain can be sent to the left, where it is put into words) and indirectly through emotion and feeling. It is quite possible, even likely, that the right brain, immersed in and responsive to emotion, responds more effectively to the emotion-charged speech of poetry than to the dry discourse of logic and rational argument. If the stumbling blocks to doing what we "know" we should lie in the right brain, then by repeating poetic words again and again, we have the chance that they will become embedded, that their message will become habit, that the right brain will become our ally in the task of doing what we ought.

It is not by mere chance that Plato said, twenty-five hundred years ago, that the cure of disease was "to be effected by the use of certain charms, and these charms are fair words by which temperance is implanted in the soul." Words have the power to move us, to make us move, to keep us on track, to give life to our deeds, especially if those words are burned into our brains through the enchanting power of poetry.

Dr. Neelon's love of poetry and his ability to recite it, laced with Rice *dieta* wisdom and soulful ponderings, really transcend description. When he weaves Mary Oliver's poem "The Journey" into Ricer testimonials and collective wisdom from a community that is sharing a common *dieta* for healing, it is a sacred experience. We all understand in the moment and in the many moments when we are held captive by his perfectly timed pauses and in the other moments when we'll recall this magic memory that we have received a profound invitation to save the only life we really can, which is our own!

Day 19: Feed Your Soul and Nurture Your Spirit through Poetry

You know that when you kindle your positive feelings, you inspire improvement in your physical health, as well as enhance and increase your neuronal connections and your power to change, so why not treat yourself to some new experiences with bibliotherapy? Whether you check out Mary Oliver's poetry books from the library (be sure to read her poem "Rice") or enjoy some of the works of

Rumi, choose one of your favorite poems and memorize it today. Similar to actively singing or playing a musical instrument, reciting a poem can be more healing than simply reading it. When we memorize a poem or know it by heart, we own the poem's truth in a deeper place; then, when we recite it to others and pay it forward, it takes us deeper yet. Check out your local paper for poetry readings in your area and attend or participate in one this month.

Poetry has been enjoyed as a conduit for change, a translator for grace, a way to express the soul's deepest longings. From David's psalms to the many New Testament miracles, anointed words have inspired our pursuit of the mystery and our understanding of why we struggle to do what we really want to do but often don't.

Sin, a Wake-Up Call to Consciousness

"For I have the desire to do what is good, but I cannot carry it out. For what I do is not the good I want to do; no, the evil I do not want to do—this I keep on doing" (Romans 7:18–19).

Many who recoil from the word *sin* may choose to replace it with a less loaded and more easily understood description for "unconscious, ignorant responses based on erroneous thinking." In other words, sin or erroneous thoughts, feelings, intentions, and beliefs cause us to miss the mark or disable us from achieving our highest calling. Given this definition, who would really want to wallow in it or, frankly, even want to go there? Although unconscious actions can often create disease, this can effectively catapult us into an awareness to become more conscious of our health and other life priorities. One of the redemptive mysteries about sin and unconscious, error-based thinking and action is that they can be a huge wake-up call and can inspire us toward consciousness and truth faster and more effectively than anything I know!

Although certain Judaic and Christian scriptures support the belief that sin can be the root cause of illness and disease (John 5:2–14), there is also scripture that says this is not true in all cases. The book of Job and many of Christ's teachings emphasize that there are many causations. Holy Scripture also contains many other nuggets of truth that can help us understand how to pursue our healings and shifts in consciousness. I'm particularly fond of Acts 3:1–10:

> One day Peter and John were going up to the temple at the time of prayer, at three in the afternoon. Now a man crippled from birth was being carried to the temple gate called Beautiful, where he was put every day to beg from those going into the temple courts. When he saw Peter and John about to enter, he asked them for money. Peter looked straight at him, as did John. Then Peter said, "Look at us!" So the man gave them his attention, expecting to get something from them. Then Peter said, "Silver or gold I do not have, but what I have I give you. In the name of Jesus Christ of Nazareth, walk." Taking him by the right hand, he helped him up, and instantly the man's feet and ankles became strong. He jumped to his feet and began to walk. Then he went with them into the temple courts, walking and jumping, and praising God.

Even those without a Christian belief system will likely find this story interesting from a psychological and quantum physics perspective. The man who was crippled from birth is invited to look up, rather than remain fixated on his handicap, and give his attention to those who are aware of their spiritual source and desirous of giving him a hand up. Whether you hear this with a Christian ear or appreciate it as an example of a quantum (physics) leap in consciousness, it is a lesson that we have all needed at some point in our lives. We need to keep our eyes raised upward, looking for our resurrective opportunities, rather than focused on our limited and scarcity-based history.

Seeking loving, mature people of God has assisted my spiritual growth and healing as much as any tool I have employed. I seek their wisdom, as well as their healing gifts.

My dear spiritual confidant Vernon Tyson elaborated, "Sin is a great separator from ourselves, our families, our environment, our roots, our fruits; it is a separator. Sin is missing the mark; it is less than the best. If you're settling for something less than the best, and that takes the center of your life, it keeps you from having the fullness that you desire to have. It's selling yourself short, which is another form of prostitution . . . selling yourself short of the health and life you most desire. There is a kind of natural force; like a rock falling, it doesn't have a mind of its own—it has force. Evil sometimes is the force of inertia, remaining on the sofa, of not doing [what we know is healthiest]; it becomes so powerful to us that it sometimes appears as if it has a mind."

Although some people may still feel uncomfortable with the words *sin* and *evil*, we all can relate to the pain and suffering that we have caused ourselves and others by making unconscious choices that have not served our higher calling. Whatever you choose to call it, when we fall into these "holes in the sidewalk" or find ourselves in places where we don't want to be, we can remember to look within for the redeeming truth. Whether it be a physical or an emotional pain, there is a root issue asking for our attention to release it. If we can approach it as an opportunity for growth, rather than as an undesired entity to resist or extinguish, this will release the resurrective potential that it was intended to teach us. Fortunately, my experience continues to assure me that as we seek love and the light, the higher calling within us all, and our knowledge of this resurrective potential in any situation, there will follow healing and miracles beyond our imaginings.

When I look back over my life, at my many unconscious, ignorant, and error-based actions, I realize that my most dramatic and significant healings, revelations in the desert, and manifestations of my dreams and goals were preceded by persistent prayers. I am assured that this loving, connecting, and creating force is eternal and will always be there for my greater good. Seeking, receiving, and sharing love and forgiveness from God, for myself and others, have also been predominant and ongoing actions in my spiritual growth and assurance.

Day 20: Our Need for Love

We all seek to be known and unconditionally loved. Because most of us get to enjoy unconditional love in the physical world only briefly, usually as newborns adored by our mothers, we naturally seek this ultimate love, on some level, for the rest of our lives. It is as if we are love-seeking missiles. Often we don't recognize this need for love and thus attempt to get this ecstasy from other substitutes, such as alcohol, drugs, our favorite comfort foods, or from relationships that had familiar vibrations or a neurotic resonance with our family of origin. Developing spiritual health and a reliable connection to the unconditional love within us is a very personal journey and is, of course, different for everyone.

A big part of my healings has been seeking and committing to relationships with others who believe in a spiritual discipline and are coming from their hearts or from the ultimate source of love and truth, thus are willing conduits. Most of the people I have sought for spiritual direction are grounded in love; they are not exempt from sin but rather seek the love of God, spend time immersed in their holy scriptures, the pursuit of truth, and prayer and have the desire to share the fullness of their hearts and pass it on.

Because I was not raised in the Catholic tradition, I did not practice confessing my sins to a spiritual elder. In fact, getting really honest with myself and others about my error-based thoughts, then my subsequent obsessive feelings, first began in an Adult Children of Alcoholics meeting. (This is a free confidential group available to people with and without faith; it is internationally renowned for assisting those with addictions of any type and is not limited to only those with alcoholic parents.) So pray to be led to a group or a spiritually mature and trustworthy person who will listen to your truth and pray for your healing.

In addition to, or in place of, a more confessional approach, you can also spend some quiet, reflective time with yourself for the same purpose. Set aside twenty minutes for spiritual reflection. You may want to start with a few minutes of centering prayer, then journalize any thoughts that surface about previous actions you performed that were unconscious, ignorant, and error-based. As you connect with your regret or shame, remember that you are communicating with the only consistent unconditionally loving

Source of Power in the Universe. You can confess directly to God, or you could ask in your journalizing for God to reveal someone to you who might become your spiritual mentor. Enjoy this time with your Creator, and co-create your spiritual healing. He or she will be glad to hear from you again!

Love and Forgive Your Enemies, Including Yourself

In a recent Lenten scriptural commentary (Luke 6:27–36), I was reminded of Jesus' commandment to love our enemies. Although I could easily imagine enemies such as Hitler or Osama bin Laden, it was really the first time that I had considered that this scripture was not only about the most obviously sinful people but about all of us, for aren't we our own worst enemies? I realized that every time I judged myself, held onto recriminations, or otherwise didn't forgive myself for some self-perceived failings, I was unwittingly getting in my own way.

This insight, that I am probably my own worst enemy, challenged me to take an inventory of things that hurt or frustrated me and events or bodily responses such as illnesses that angered or annoyed me. Then I needed to consider whether I viewed these as my enemies and fought them, or viewed them as my teachers, providing an invitation and an opportunity for spiritual growth and healing. I recalled how much internal struggle I had felt with my out-of-control emotional attachment to resentment; despite my desire and prayers to stop doing what I knew was hurting me more than it was anyone else, I felt addicted to it. It was a deeply ingrained habit and response to any situation in which I felt that an authority figure was trying to impede my freedom or restrict my opinion. This process led me to remember the last act of my healing story.

Prior to the weekend of my spiritual and emotional healing from the root cause of my crippling joint disorder, I had spent nine months intensifying my desire to be totally healed and whole. I had been seeking God and people who I felt were filled with His or Her power. I had acted as if I would be healed—despite the fact that there were no physical signs of this in sight. I sought out and benefited from many positive and empowering sources, from mind, body, and spirit healing books to prayer partners and confessors, to healing conferences. And I exercised what I learned; I resumed an inner healing practice of meditation, yoga, and journalizing.

As you may remember from chapter 3, where I summarized how Dr. Wally Purcell led us through the emotional inventory and exploration, this experience was a powerful way to align my thoughts, feelings, and spiritual expectancy, thus readying myself for the healing of my resentment. (To refresh your memory, Wally asked us to write down any emotion that we felt we were struggling with: to write about an emotion that was not serving our higher calling, to pinpoint when it became apparent, and to describe what we planned to do about it.) When we completed the exercise, Wally asked whether anyone wanted to role-play his or her emotion with him, and he chose me as the most enthusiastic, or possibly desperate, participant. Although I had never participated in a role-playing session before, Wally quickly threw a few fast hardballs my way, and I realized that this process was not necessarily going to be fun. Wally, role-playing my resentment, quickly and coldly said, "I've been around since you were eight years old, and if you didn't want me around, I wouldn't still be here." I immediately realized I was in for a tough game. Approximately forty-five minutes later, in front of about forty people, we ended with him asking, "What do you want from me?" And I whimpered, "Peace."

After a closing prayer, I drove home. Although I was emotionally exhausted and still in physical pain, I definitely felt that something deep inside of me had shifted. It was not until the next morning when I was driving back to the retreat center, on an interstate, that I realized just how different I felt inside. I spotted my boss's car ahead of me. She was the one person whom I had habitually resented the most during the previous decade. Of course, I had some justifiable reasons, right? Although she had done numerous, totally unacceptable acts, such as moving my office while I was on vacation, it was certainly not healing my joints to continue to dwell on my litany of her personal shortcomings. But what was so amazing was the intensity of the contraction I felt around my heart area when I first saw her car. I felt the walls leap up around my heart as I began to emotionally defend myself from her.

I remember thinking, I can pretend that I didn't see her car, and I'll just drive by her, and she'll never know that I saw her. The armorlike pressure around my heart was intense and startling, similar to what I imagine a heart attack would feel like. As soon as my car caught up with hers, the armor around my heart miraculously melted. I was instantly overwhelmed by the unconditional love of God for her, for me, for all of the people in the world who allow their mental and emotional baggage to separate them from the love and unity that are available to us all. It was physically the most profound miracle of my life! As I readied myself to beep the horn and started to wave excitedly, I realized that it was not even her!

To have my heart blasted open at eight in the morning, simply by driving up alongside a car that I mistakenly thought was being driven by someone I had resented was really mind-bending! Mixed with my spiritual elation was the sobering realization that if I had put my body through that much stress over a car that merely looked like my boss's car, how much unnecessary damage, pain, and suffering must I be creating on a regular basis due to my ignorant and ego-driven state? When I really became aware of the self-inflicted pain that I created with my unconscious and erroneous thoughts, and then I connected with all of the other people in the world who are unconsciously creating what they do not really want with their mistaken thoughts and unhealthy emotional responses— it felt like Yom Kippur combined with Easter! It was a profound moment. This much clarity and awareness of human suffering and the power within us to resurrect it were worth my nine months of crippling pain.

When I drove up to the retreat center's entrance, planning to run to tell Wally what had happened, he was waiting on the front porch. He first asked how I was feeling and explained that I would at some point experience resentment again, but I would notice that the *intent* of it had changed. I laughed out loud and told him that

I had already had Resentment Change 101 class on the way over and described what had happened to me on my morning commute. We laughed and celebrated the creative ways the Spirit manifests and how comical this often is!

Although I had prayed for approximately nine months to hear confirmation from within about leaving my job, about a week after this deep healing experience I awoke from a dream that told me that today was the day to give notice. I asked my boss for an afternoon appointment with her, where I lovingly told her that I would be leaving and that I needed to share with her a bit about everything I had learned. I felt no resentment but instead love and mercy.

Despite the fact that I was still in physical pain, it was clear to me that she also had much unrealized pain, and I truly hoped that she could benefit from our relationship, at least a fraction of what I had gained. By the end of our appointment we were both in tears, as I learned that she was an adult child of alcoholic parents and that she struggled with a control addiction but did not really know how to heal herself. As I left work that day, I knew that my healing was eminent. I desired it with all of my being. I had tenaciously sought God for direction, timing, and truth, and I did my best to act as I felt, led by the Spirit. The prescription was ideal, the timing divine, and my healing inevitable. Within the week, without my lifting a finger to make a phone call to seek out other employment opportunities, I had received the ultimate consulting offer from a hospital in Texas. Oh yes, and the same week all of my joint pain went away! After nine months of pain, struggle, fear, and faith building, multiplied by thousands of times, I felt as if I were truly showered with blessings beyond my imaginings. Yes, that was a very good week! Hallelujah!

Healing Is a Community and Family Affair

Disease and healing can build community like no other life experiences I have known. At the Rice Diet Program, we regularly get to witness and be part of participants' spiritual shifts in consciousness and their resulting physical healings. All of us humans seem to learn and then relearn lessons many times, on many levels, during our healing journeys. At the Rice Diet Program or any place or time when we slow down and look within, we open up more easily to such awakenings and to other people. Although it is often easier for us to see a spiritually connecting thread or a life lesson in illnesses or tragedies that befall others, rather than in our own lives when we are in the midst of our own trials, it is enriching and rewarding at those times to be surrounded by trusted fellow sojourners whose spiritual maturity we have confidence in.

While Anna Marie credits the Rice Diet with saving her life, she has been a spiritual beacon for countless others whose lives we've shared. Anna Marie is one of the most loving friends and fellow Ricers I know and is herself profoundly blessed with a gift of healing. Like many other people with that gift, she has suffered numerous dramatic health crises and healings of her own. In the process, she has learned to prioritize her own health needs in order to receive the miracles she so generously facilitates for many others. She categorizes her specific needs into those that are physical (a very-low-sodium diet), emotional, and spiritual (creating time for her mind and heart to commune with her Creator for her own benefit, as well as for others'). Her comical and creative way of describing her faith is contagious, as you'll see below!

> Someone once said, "Miracles are only miracles because we don't believe they can happen." I believe that often crisis speaks God's design to increase our faith and belief in possibilities. I am a miracle, and I know angels dwell among us. On December 26, 1997, my whole world was turned upside down! It was my birthday. I knew I was tired. I thought it was due to a heavy lecture schedule in Venezuela the week before Christmas. I was wrong. My heart stopped that day in the mountains of Virginia. The rescue squad had been called and responded accordingly. I was transported to Augusta General, breaking speed limits in an ice storm. I don't remember anything but a feeling of slipping away . . . even peace.

I was awake and alert three days later in intensive care. I was asked by a team of doctors, "Mrs. Hancock, who is the president of the U.S.?" I commented with a giggle, "Everyone knows that's Hillary Clinton!" My husband said, "She's back!" My experience with good health was short-lived . . . long enough to eat a slice of that birthday cake, and I was back in the hospital. For the next year I would experience many hospitals and many emergency rooms. As I worsened, a countless number of physicians indicated I could not live much longer . . . maybe a few weeks. The irony is that my husband, Tommy, developed the specialty of hospital law in the U.S., and he is one of the founders and CEO of Diamond Health Care Corporation. He owned hospitals, but none could help or save me. I, who lectured on faith, prepared to die. When I finally took to the bed with legs too weak to perform and speech too garbled to understand, I was convinced the end was near. I did everything but *die*. I was ready, but God wasn't.

Who could believe the Rice Diet saved my life? Who could believe that all the medicine in the world couldn't? I was on a strict regimen of rice and fruit. Liquid potassium was introduced as I couldn't swallow pills. In two weeks' time I was walking and back to my babbling brook self! There are many who still can't accept that a nutrition regimen saved my life. I continue ten years later with rice and fruit and potassium, plus grains, beans, vegetables, some meat, and other unprocessed, no-salt-added foods—and I am well! I am enjoying three grandchildren, have seen my younger daughter married and give birth—I have seen new life and have my own back! Miracles are only miracles because we don't believe they can happen. They happen every day. It is God's will. The Rice Diet Program is a well of healing love available to all of us and, I believe, designed by God Himself with the help of earth angels.

Dreams, a Door to Knowing
God and Ourselves

My appreciation and understanding of dreams were greatly enhanced by the friendship and teachings of Morton Kelsey, who was a psychologist, a teacher, an Episcopalian priest, and the author of more than twenty books. Although it has long been accepted that dreams are like doors to unconscious parts of the human psyche, his studies with the Swiss psychologist Carl Jung led him to understand that these unconscious places can be avenues for divine inspiration. In addition to his keen intellect, he had an ethereal, yet practical way of helping you connect to the unconditional love and wisdom of the Divine. He understood that the unconscious is where God first touches us, and he was incredibly gifted in encouraging us to carefully listen to our dreams and translate these revelations into our everyday lives.

After a brief evening introduction at his "Healing with Dreams" conference, Morton Kelsey and his friend Tommy Tyson prayed that we would be blessed with dreams of revelation. I awoke the following morning with the most magical and intense dream of my life. The dream was in Technicolor, and I was walking along an amazingly idyllic forest path, through an antique covered bridge carpeted with plush tapestry fabric, complete with artistically designed cabinets and cubbies containing every imaginable art supply. Then I entered a grotesque scene that was very unsettling. Although still disturbed by the dream's finale, I knew that the dream had significance, so, during the break, I hurried to seek Morton's opinion of my dream. He listened carefully to all of the glorious, then startling details, and with more compassion, grace, and acceptance than I have ever witnessed, he smiled and said that he thought I had received an invitation from God to explore my darker side! He proceeded to say that God knows me the best and has invited me to know more of myself. Because I was still unaware that I had a darker side, I shared this with him, and he gently responded,

"We all do!" Never has anyone so lovingly suggested that another seek therapy! It was as if he was giving me a very special gift when he explained that "a good therapist can often help us explore and learn more about ourselves." The very next week I met a wonderful therapist who proved Morton's words to be true.

Carl Jung believed that dreams communicate with us through the rich language of symbols. And because most modern men and women have forgotten how to think in symbols, Jung's gift has been a significant one. He taught us that by paying attention to our dreams and the symbols they contain, we can gain access to a new and deeper realm that can bring balance to our conscious view. Dr. Ira Progoff also did work with Carl Jung and thus had a wonderful grasp of the importance of dreams. Then Progoff translated his understanding into a simple, accessible, and profoundly revealing method of interpreting our significant dreams.

The Progoff Intensive Journal program is well worth the weekend investment, and although it is nearly impossible to condense, I will nonetheless offer the briefest summary of his method for dream interpretation: Keep a journal by your bed, and write out the full dream as soon as you awaken from it. Then on the left-hand margin of a piece of paper, list all of the words in the dream that are not articles (the words *a, an,* or *the*); next, immediately write to the right of each of these words the first word that comes to your mind; then read the original word from the dream again, and write in a second column, on the same line, the next word that comes to your mind; and again return to the original word and write a third word that comes to your mind. Do this for all of the words from your dream, then go back and read the three words that you have written for each dream word, one at a time, and circle the one that has the most resonance or feels best to you. After you have done this for all of the words, you simply read down the list of circled words, which, after all, are symbols for the dream's meaning. The first time I did this, it absolutely blew my mind! Now I admit that when I have done it, it was not a letter-perfect translation, but very rarely are the insights revealed not worth the effort. Obviously, this takes a bit of time, so I do this only with dreams that I think are significant for me.

Although many people may think that they don't dream, they simply don't remember their dreams. We all dream. If you believe that we can experience God and the realm of the Spirit, then dreams may be one of the most common avenues through which God communicates. Many of the world's religions have maintained that humans can experience God; from Judaism to Christianity, to Islam, Hinduism, Zoroastrianism, and the Chinese folk religions, we find in each one the contention that we can come into contact with God. They all have developed methods of prayer to achieve this contact. Throughout the Old and the New Testament, stories describe how God approached human beings through visions, dreams, voices in the wilderness, and a variety of other unique ways.

In Morton Kelsey's book *Dreams: A Way to Listen to God*, he summarized his theological and historical perspective on our openness to dreams as a means to communicate with the Divine. He stated that "Jesus also introduced two completely new ideas. He taught that we may call upon this power that rules the universe and may address this very power that staggers our imagination with the word 'Abba'," which means 'Daddy'." He went on to say, "The second idea Jesus introduced was that *the Kingdom of God is within us and among us*." He elaborated that in addition to God manifesting through dreams, healings, miracles, and prophecies, Jesus and his followers were convinced that Abba, if sought like a daddy, wanted to actually reveal Himself to those who turned to Him in sincerity and silence. He explained that Christian philosophies of the last 350 years have often overlooked or minimized the fact that our Creator wants to come into contact with us, and that we can actually know this God. He also briefly described how a "division arose between the Church (who didn't want her authority questioned) and the secular world because the Church refused to tolerate, let alone encourage, the sort of scientific thought that allowed humans to discover that the earth revolves around the sun. The church's intolerance of this inquiring spirit forced scientific thought to develop on a completely secular level and to become antireligious to the point of maintaining that human beings have no

Godly spirit. This narrow-minded attitude eventually caused thinking Christians to adopt secular thought exclusively and become convinced that God could be known only through reason and not through experience." So many have continued to put God in the "heaven or somewhere else" box and have come to believe that they cannot expect to have a personal experience of, or with, God. Remember the quantum physics lesson "We get what we think, feel, and believe is possible"? Well, why not practice what previous centuries of spiritually alive believers have? If you desire and seek God and people who are connected with the Creator and act as if you expect this intimate spiritual connection to occur, it will build a foundation on which your experience of knowing will grow.

I have had my most powerful, revealing dreams before and during the greatest, most pivotal turning points in my life. The overwhelmingly obvious confirmation that the Creator is at the helm of my life has carried me through every major leap I have made. When I was eighteen years old, I awoke in the middle of the night, knowing that my daddy had just died of a heart attack. Despite the fact that he was only fifty years old and no one had had any warning that he was sick, I dreamed, or at least awoke knowing, that he had just died. I don't know whether it was a dream or I was simply awakened by his departing spirit, but I was so sure, I telephoned him in the middle of the night. The unanswered call and the coroner's report the next day confirmed his time of death. I also dreamed the date that I would be reunited with my husband. I believe this was God's grace so that I could bear the next nine months of a broken engagement before we were married. In addition, I dreamed the actual birth date of my only niece, which gave me blessed assurance of her healthy delivery, despite her forty-three-year-old mother's previous four miscarriages in two years.

As I recall the many intimate and loving connections that I have experienced with my Creator through dreams, I realize why I felt compelled to include them here. Dreams have been one of the, if not *the*, most profound pathways for my divine revelations. One day I raced over to see my spiritual mentor, Tommy Tyson, to share my ecstasy of awakening with a profound, prophetic dream.

Tommy gave me a sly, impish grin and ingeniously responded, "If we don't listen to God when we're awake, He'll come to us when we are asleep!" When these dreams come, I know that what has been revealed will occur. If I continue to walk toward the prize, it is a done deal!

Some of you may not currently remember your dreams, but I can assure you that the following techniques can greatly enhance your ability to retain them more often. First, desire to remember them and begin to anticipate and expect them. Second, seek God and the company of those who you feel are mature in their faith, read books such as Morton Kelsey's *Dreams: A Way to Listen to God*, and attend conferences that include dream work, such as Progoff's Intensive Journal Process. Although I have never met anyone who can program their dreams effectively on a daily basis, nor do I think we necessarily know enough to benefit from such a practice, I have found that God provides such personal revelation when I am most desirous and in need of it.

Someone once said, "Expect the best and you often get it!" I have seen this to be true in my own life and in the lives of many people I have served and shared with. While facilitating classes, I often encourage participants to take off their imaginary lids, hats, helmets, and visors and make a dream list of what they have always wanted to do regardless of how "out there" their critical brain may at first judge this process to be. Despite the fact that we are all quite practiced at making up stories that justify why we cannot do certain things or cannot actualize our wildest dreams, let's play the angel's advocate. You can benefit from such a dream experiential in the comfort of your bed at home.

Day 21: Intentionally Inspiring Rest and Creating Desired Dreams

Tonight perform the following preparatory acts to inspire a deep and restful sleep and to have a desired dream, remember it, and document it for further reflection. To relax yourself, you can meditate in your favorite way. If you have not become practiced or comfortable with mindfulness meditation, you can get your mind to a calm alpha-wavelength state simply by counting down from ten to one, over the course of three to four deep breaths. If you visualize these numbers in your mind's eye while you count down, with your eyes closed, and remind yourself to relax more with each number counted, you will be very relaxed by the time you reach number one. Some high-strung people may find it easier to count themselves down, rather than simply notice their thoughts. I think many people may find that the counting approach gives them something concrete to do as they calm their mind and relax into the alpha state.

Once you are deeply relaxed, ask God to reveal what your next mission or divine plan will be. You may also use this experience to request a revelation of God's will in a matter of concern. You may journal to God at this time, or, if you prefer to stay still, you may suggest to yourself that you will have a dream revealing the answer to a problem you have struggled with lately. You could simply state, with assuredness, that you will dream about the learning opportunities that are available in a recent area of concern or interest and tell yourself that you will remember the dream on waking. It's important to have physical confirming aids to psychologically assist this spoken intention, so before you lie down, place a full glass of water, your journal, a pen, and a reading light beside your bed. One Ricer said that she preferred documenting her dreams by speaking near a voice-activated tape recorder so that she could more easily return to sleep if she needed. After you have stated or written down your desired intention to dream, drink half of the glass of water and calmly affirm your goal by stating or praying, "I want to dream about what I should do about . . . and I will dream of God's revelation concerning this issue." Go to sleep expecting to hear from your Creator and to finish the other half glass of water in the morning.

The Power of the Woods

The woods have long been one of my favorite environments for spiritual renewal. Of course, as a child I did not choose to surround myself with trees for health reasons. I wanted to be in the woods to gather materials to build forts, to swing from vines, and to conquer the ultimate walkie-talkie tag challenge (our middle school version of hide-and-seek using walkie-talkies to direct or taunt the seeker). Although you may not have the upper-body strength or the burning desire to get your exercise through swinging from vines and playing tag, you certainly may become inspired to walk through the woods more often, especially after reading the latest research on forest bathing. *Shinrin-yoku* is a word that was coined in 1982 by the Forestry Agency of the Japanese government to encourage the enhancement of physical and mental health. It is a compound word made up of words that mean "forest" and "bathing" and was probably designed to convey, as with sea bathing, the potential curative or therapeutic effect of immersing oneself in the forest's atmosphere and terrain.

For decades we have been enticed by interesting research on the health benefits of a natural environment, but we have just scratched the surface of understanding how deeply we are indebted to nature and the multisensory advantages of living close to the natural world. Simply the *sight* of nature really matters to your health. Roger S. Urlich's clinical trials, conducted in 1984, which examined the recovery records of hospital patients for ten years, found that patients with tree views had shorter hospitalizations than did patients with brick-wall views.

From studies dealing with the five senses separately, Yoshifumi Miyazaki and others' research clarified that simply the *smell* of Japanese cedar wood lowered blood pressure and regional cerebral blood flow in the prefrontal area, and Riho Mishima and colleagues' research found that the *sound* of murmuring water lowered blood pressure as well. Although some studies evaluated the effects of longer periods of forest exposure, these last two cited studies by Miyazaki and Mishima showed that experiencing health benefits did not take long: the changes in physiological parameters caused by inhaling the odor of wood or hearing the sound of murmuring water were observed within sixty to ninety seconds. Japanese scientists have hard evidence that walking in the forest decreases blood glucose levels of diabetic patients, and that people who viewed forest scenery versus urban settings had a 13 percent lower blood concentration of the stress hormone cortisol. Forest walking versus city walking boosted the activity of T cells, which are immune cells that fight cancer. These scientists also reported that people living near forested areas, when compared to those not living near forests, had lower mortality rates for cancers of the prostate, breast, lung, uterus, kidney, and colon.

Jennifer Ackerman has written a beautiful article titled "Breathing Trees," available through the Wilderness Society (www.wilderness .org). I urge you to visit this Web site, subscribe to the newsletter, and request the back issue featuring Ackerman's article. Her wonderful article and gracious referral to this research were another healing-at-the-roots experience. She wrote about researchers who analyzed air samples in the Sierra forest and could identify only 70 of the 120 compounds they found. While the Japanese researchers believe that inhaling phytoncides, essential wood oils emitted by plants, is partly responsible for the boosted activity of the T cells and that two other woody compounds, alpha-pinene and borneol, likely help us reduce our fatigue, these are but a fraction of the many reasons for us to be grateful for trees.

I love how Jennifer Ackerman intimately described our symbiotic relationship with plants: "When we inhale forest air, some of these molecules ride the currents into our lungs and there pass into our bloodstream to affect our cells. . . . I love this notion that plant molecules speak to human cells, revealing as it does that deep common kinship of living things long known by poets." She quoted George Herbert, who wrote, "Herbs gladly cure our flesh, because that they / Find their acquaintance there."

I also felt a kinship with Ackerman when she expressed her concern for our ignorance of the unseen components of forest ecology and "the range of interlocking links in ecological webs that make predicting the effects of habitat destruction such a tricky business. When I think that we are losing forests at a rate of seven million hectares a year, and with them, who knows how many pinenes and phytoncides, known and unknown, with potential to ease our stress and heal our bodies, I feel a black wave of despair." She, too, ended on a hopeful note. We can save the trees, the planet, and our health, but it will require a major and rapid growth spurt in our awareness.

Day 22: The Shinrin-Yoku Challenge

This *Shinrin-yoku*, or forest bathing, experiential will be one of the fastest and most obvious beneficial responses you will create through your Rice *dieta* immersion. All you have to do is find the nearest wooded area or park and enjoy your one hour of aerobic exercise there twice within this week. Then in the exercise and feeling sections of your *Dieta* Journal note any improvements in your mood, clarity of thought, and gratitude to nature. Consider participating in local events that would benefit the environment, such as Earth Day walks or runs. Perhaps join the Sierra Club or another organization that sponsors educational hikes to provide a new, active resource to support your personal and environmental health interests.

Spend more time outside and with nature in general and cultivate your connectedness and gratitude to our life- and health-giving planet. Last month, my son and I went gleaning, a practice described in the Old Testament, where one collects the remaining foods yet to be harvested from a field. In addition to our burning a couple of hundred calories with other generous folks, my son learned the age-old joy of performing community service in the great outdoors.

A Personal Love for Nature

My appreciation for nature and my love for trees extends back as far as I can remember. This relationship with trees grew exponentially when I was in my early twenties and the thrill and allure of climbing 300-foot fir trees to pick their cones for reforestation while camping in the woods and making $200 to $400 per day with a cooperative called Hoedads was too enticing to refuse. A friend who invited me to join him on this adventure assured me that I could get over my fear of heights by climbing a 50-foot fir tree the first day, a 100-foot one the next day, then a 150-foot one the following day, and by the end of the week I'd be laughing at the top of a 300-footer. I was crazy enough to take the dare and proved him right. We had a blast, and after three months of climbing trees daily and enjoying northern California and Oregon vistas, we were in the best shape any of us had ever known, plus we thought we were rich!

Those adventures are a book unto themselves, but reading Richard Preston's *The Wild Trees: A Story of Passion and Daring* took me back to those thrilling days and to truths about tree roots and life, which have sustained me physically, metaphysically, and spiritually without my full knowledge of that which is not physically seen yet grounds me and connects me with others, thus empowering me to live my life with passion. Preston wrote, "A redwood tree sits on a flat pancake of roots, spreading in all directions away from the tree. A redwood has no taproot. A taproot is a strong, vertical root, shaped like a carrot, that stabs straight down under a tree and acts as an anchor, helping to keep the tree upright. The pancake of roots under a redwood spreads out and narrows down into a fine, dense mat of threads no more than about two feet thick. These fine roots extend outward for unknown distances from the tree, perhaps a hundred yards or more. They eventually merge with the threadlike roots of other redwoods, forming a tangled mat of roots. The roots of a redwood forest resemble a pad made of felt. The pad seems to support all the redwoods that are in a stand; they are all anchored by the common mat."

To fathom how a 2-foot, or less, deep mat of fine threadlike roots can hold a 370-foot redwood for more than a thousand years rocks our rational minds. Fortunately, the power of the supportive network for humans is equally beyond our comprehension. So let's bring these lofty truths from trees down to earth to assist us in manifesting the fruits we are here to produce. Our passionate potential and supportive network can be realized and renewed via a multitude of practices, and creating a map to remind us of our goals, dreams, and course can be one of the most effective ways of harnessing them and grounding us.

Diagramming Your Dream via a PERT Chart, Conceptual Mapping, or Growing Your Tree

Diagramming and mapping strategies help people identify and address the what, why, when, where, and how to manifest their desires and goals. Because most of us are visually oriented and procrastinators by nature, it really is a powerful tool to see how we might imagine getting from our present point A to where we want to go, point B. Engineering types may prefer the diagramming and mapping approaches to growing their tree, so both will be described and illustrated for you to practice. Then you can choose the one that most appeals to you.

I was introduced to the Program Evaluation and Review Technique, or PERT, charting by my brother about fifteen years ago, as we discussed my many imagined challenges of writing my first book and getting it published. He said that practically all businesspeople have PERT charts, which outline and connect strategies to get any big project off the ground and to help them brainstorm about its preferred process and direction. You map out each of the known steps that are necessary to accomplish the end product, by organizing needed actions into arenas (departments), sequencing, and dating the specified actions' completion. When we adopted this technique for Ricers at the Rice Diet Program, it evolved to address all of the dimensions of our lives that needed attention.

These charts can be designed any way your brain is inspired to create them, but I often illustrate mine by putting a circle, approximately two inches in diameter, in the middle of the page that identifies the goal. My first book was titled *Heal Your Heart*, so that was in the middle circle of my PERT chart. Then I drew straight lines out from the circle, with each of these lines denoting, or serving as the axis for, arenas to be addressed. My first line held "all major, direct actions needed to have a book published." To hold this many specifics, I drew lines at right angles off this line, then labeled actions in sequence, and stated the completion dates.

My offshoot lines specified actions to do in this order:

Go to library to find books that list all New York City book agents, 1/10/94

Go to New York City to interview and hire an agent, 2/6/94

Complete book, 3/29/94

Write letter and send manuscript to family friend with publishing connection, 4/2/94

A different spoke that came off the center circle specified the emotional and spiritual support that needed my attention: pray with mentor, Tommy Tyson, regarding my sense that John Wiley & Sons was to be the publishing house that bought this book, 1/19/94; attend Tommy's conferences and spiritually supportive community network, with dates for plans already made. Another spoke contained my physical disciplines: to walk, practice yoga, and so on.

Although most PERT charts are dream or ideal trajectories that are proposed, and life does not always go as we plan, this process does help us get more clear about our priorities, how to organize our lives to manifest our goals, what to delegate, when to seek supportive assistance, and basically how to empower ourselves to complete our mission. I have never had a PERT chart that was actualized as accurately as this first one was initially projected. At that time I knew absolutely nothing about publishing, except that I thought John Wiley & Sons was the most respected publishing house in the world, but I asked Tommy Tyson (my spiritual mentor of more than a decade) to pray that the book be sold to Wiley. This publisher was my only offer! PERT and mapping charts are not guaranteed Christmas lists, but they can be very revealing when we prayerfully consider and contemplate our visions for what we feel may be our next calling or heart's desire. Who knows? This practice may totally revamp your definition of miraculous!

Why not fully participate in actualizing the exciting dreams and visions you have previously only toyed with or played lip service to? Remember, the equation for manifesting is: desire + seek + act = co-create.

So pick up your paper and pencil and complete this PERT, mapping, or tree-based game-planning experiential!

Day 23: Make a PERT Chart or Prune and Pursue Your Spiritual Health Tree

Any method that you like and will use to envision and inspire your pursuits and purpose is the best choice for you. Because it calls to you, you will be much more likely to use it and grow with it. Diagram the dimensions of your life that need attention to manifest the dreams you envision. This road map will help you distill your deepest longings and ground your lofty dreams to become manifested realities. If you prefer to visualize your upcoming growth with your tree's roots and branches, please do so. Either method will be helpful; the format is simply a personal preference.

I have described and illustrated many pathways to enhance your spiritual health. You may find this refresher section a convenient source to help you determine the supportive roots and branches you most need to practice to co-create your goals and dreams:

- Meditation (from mindfulness meditations, loving-kindness meditations, and HeartMath techniques to centering prayer and walking meditations)
- Spiritual and religious disciplines (prayer groups, Bible studies, and 12-step groups)
- Introspective and energy-moving practices (yoga, tai chi, dance)
- Expressive writing and journalizing with your nondominant hand
- Dream suggestions (to inspire and enhance dream retention)
- Massage, EFT, and other energy work (axiatonal therapy, breath work, laying on of hands; there's more in chapter 7)

- Seek musically inspired revelations (from Gregorian chants to "Wind Beneath My Wings" by Bette Midler and "One Chance," performed by Paul Potts on *Britain's Got Talent*, a talent show similar to *America's Got Talent*).
- Exercise your renewed spirit by volunteering with soup kitchens, farmers' markets, the Society for St. Andrew's, or other like-minded organizations.

PART TWO

A Deeper Sense of
True Health

6

Conscious Consumption

*What holds true for the soil—that you must give it more
than you take away—also holds true for nations, institutions,
marriage, friendship, education, in short for human culture
as a whole.*
—Robert Pogue Harrison

Our health usually flourishes when our thoughts, feelings, and beliefs are in alignment with our life choices and when our actions are grounded in integrity and are consistent with our ideals and convictions. As we move into the twenty-first century and become increasingly aware of how our cultural unconsciousness and overconsumption have greatly endangered our health and our environment, we have also become empowered to make better, more conscious, life-sustaining choices and decisions. The power of this truth became crystal clear to me, my family, and everyone at the Rice Diet Program during the last couple of years when we experienced a radical reawakening to the connection between what we put into our mouths and how we live our lives.

In 2008, my two colleagues—a fellow dietitian and an intern— and I had the enormous pleasure of attending a conference with about 750 farmers from the Carolinas. The conference was orga- nized by the Carolina Farm Stewardship Association, a nonprofit organization committed to promoting sustainable agriculture in the Carolinas by inspiring, educating, and organizing farmers, as well as consumers. Although all three of us were semivegetarians and quite interested in the locally grown, organic food movement, we wanted to extend our embrace beyond the raised-bed herb garden that we had created a year earlier at the Rice Diet Program.

The profundity of that weekend's effect on us may be hard for you to fully imagine, given the fact that I have been eating a whole foods diet for thirty-five years and have often eaten organic foods during this time, but the conference provided me with a new lens through which to view my food and the food of my fellow Ricers. To share food, community, and our mutual commitment to grow and provide the highest-quality food, for health and environmental reasons, to consumers who were geographically nearby truly engen- dered a head- and heart-opening epiphany. These 750-plus farmers were the most committed community I had ever encountered. Their common denominators were that they cared about producing high- quality food, enhancing the health of their land, and promoting one another's success. They came with open minds and hearts to learn and share with others.

Together, bonded by our mutual priorities and vision, we all lis- tened attentively to our keynote speaker, organic watchdog leader Mark Kastel, the cofounder of the Cornucopia Institute. Then we bonded further with the farmers who were selling their heirloom seeds in the hall, as they proudly shared stories of whose grand- mother or friend had bequeathed them the treasured seeds. When I handled these precious seeds, while knowing how agribusiness has limited our seed varieties so radically, I had a multisensory flashback to my childhood, when seed varieties actually produced foods with unique and special flavors, smells, and textures. These people were committed to a holy work, a mitzvah-filled career. The attendees seemed akin to what I imagine members of the early church were like: they were excited to help and share with one another, everything from their time to their tractors!

The farmer who received the grandest award was the one who had saved his family farm from bankruptcy and had turned the corner in his efforts to co-create a sustainable agricultural endeavor. I realized that the local organic movement, a key wake-up call to save our food supply and global resources (land, water, air quality), mirrored our nation's need to heal at the root other major health issues, such as dealing with epidemics of chronic disease. This intensive weekend experience, filled with new information and fueled by feelings that regenerated me in the core of my being, sent us back home with a fresh passion and enthusiasm for the many ways we could walk our talk.

We returned to the Rice Diet Program and shared our experience with my husband, Bob, who was simultaneously being energized by Michael Pollan's *The Omnivore's Dilemma* and Jane Goodall's *The Harvest of Hope*. We quickly committed to buying and serving as much organic food as our seasonal and geographical priorities would allow. Ricers who had previously never tried organic foods were raving about them. Soon thereafter, we were vermi-composting vegetarian scraps from our kitchen, showing the film *The Future of Food* monthly, and sharing the latest knowledge that our farmer friends had imparted to us.

Due in part to this inspiring information, Bob has lost more than forty pounds, attaining his optimal weight for the first time in more than twenty years. I believe that a more important reason he succeeded in achieving his desired weight this time, compared to the dozens of earlier times when he did not, can be traced to two deeper motives.

I believe Bob's passion to pursue his goal weight was ignited one Sunday night several years ago when our ten-year-old's words of wisdom left him speechless. After Bob wallowed in his frustration and regret about another weekend of overeating good Italian food and overdrinking red wine, he promised himself that he was going on the Rice Diet tomorrow! Our son said, "Dad, no offense or anything, but when you say that, I don't believe you anymore." Bob heard our son's heartfelt words, and Bob's desire to do what he said he was going to do took a quantum leap. I think he was motivated not only to achieve his optimal weight but also to set an example for our son to be true to his word, to actually do what he said—not to habitually say one thing and do another.

Maintaining his optimal weight had not previously eluded Bob due to a lack of knowledge of, or experience with, needed lifestyle changes for health promotion and disease prevention. In addition to being at the top of his Andover class, a Yale University honors graduate, and then a standout at Duke Medical School, he went on to envision and develop the first and largest cardiac data bank in the world. His desire to create the cardiac data bank was primarily inspired by his early belief that cardiac bypass surgery, although relieving symptoms initially, would not necessarily prolong a heart patient's life or reduce his or her chance of having future heart attacks. (Bob's intuition continues to be proved true more than three decades later, as is documented in numerous major studies and review articles; note the 2008 Mayo Clinic Proceedings and the 2009 *American Journal of Cardiology* articles in the reference section.) Bob, inspired by a preventive approach over surgical intervention, became the medical director of the largest cardiac rehabilitation center in the United States, then worked beside Dr. Walter Kempner, the founder of the world-renowned Duke University Rice Diet Program, for more than nine years before he was entrusted with its direction in 1992. Bob and many other learned dieters have come to realize that the business of weight loss and maintenance is not solely a left-brained operation, as he explains below.

> I have always said that losing weight and taking care of ourselves is not an intellectual process. As far as weight loss is concerned, we all know what to do. Eat less and exercise more. We behave as we feel. In other words, our feelings are what cause our behavior, not our intellects. If we repeat any behavior over and over again, that behavior becomes us. We

feel comfortable with that behavior and uncomfortable with alternate behaviors.

Recently, I have managed to get my weight back down to my high school weight and improve my overall health. This effort was inspired by what I learned about food from reading Michael Pollan's books (*The Omnivore's Dilemma: A Natural History of Four Meals* and *In Defense of Food: An Eater's Manifesto*) and Jane Goodall's book *Harvest for Hope: A Guide to Mindful Eating*. I now eat local and organic. If I do eat meat (other than seafood) and I occasionally do, it has to be from an animal raised on its natural diet, not corn, even if it is organic corn. Dairy products must be from cows raised on pasture and eggs from real free-range chickens (not just chickens that are raised with access to free range). I don't eat anything containing high-fructose corn syrup or GM corn or its by-products. On this diet, I eat well, take care of myself, my family, the plants and animals, and the earth.

This sounds as if an intellectual process (learning about food) had caused the change in my behavior. But it hadn't. What had happened was that this new knowledge made me so angry that I decided not to play in their game. I have always been a little paranoid. Then I went through the "Yeah, but that doesn't mean they're not out to get me" stage. But with this new knowledge about what is going on in the food industry, I finally realized that I'm just collateral damage. They don't even know I'm here. I could now take the energy provided by my anger and channel it into a behavioral change. This behavioral change was caused by a powerful emotion: anger.

From my perspective, Bob's change in thinking, eating, and being came about by tapping into his passion or true heart's desire. He was then able to make a quantum leap in his awareness of what he wanted to eat versus what he had been eating—in other words, truly desiring to eat whole foods that are preferably organic and locally grown because they are healthiest, rather than GM-corn-fed animals and disease-promoting, environment-polluting foods that evolved due to the greed of agribusinessmen and politicians. Passion and consciousness are two very powerful places to come from. When we awaken to, and live with, the understanding that every choice we make in our lives can come either from passion and consciousness or from indifference and habit, we have entered the arena where we can heal at the roots of the lives we have thus far created. We all have the freedom to choose consciously or to react or respond habitually without true awareness—in this present moment and in the next moment.

Actualizing and maintaining the weight, health, and lives we desire requires a *dieta*, a lifestyle that nurtures our physical, mental, emotional, and spiritual needs. To heal at this level requires examining each aspect of all that sustains us—of everything that we consume, from our new insistence on eating organic, locally grown foods, to consciously choosing literature, arts, and communities that empower our senses and inspire us to actualize our true purpose in life.

What Are We Consuming?

In many ways, it comes down to our becoming aware of and responsible for what we consume—from the food on our plates to the fuel in our cars, to the lifestyle choices that affect our bodies, our neighborhoods, and our planet. There are many, many levels of awakening to our consumption, but we'll primarily hone in on our *consumption of food, consumption of natural resources*, and *how we spend our time*, three of the most valued and influential commodities in our honest pursuit of integrity. Although these categories overlap in many complex ways, focusing on them will help us get a handle on this multifaceted, complicated, and insatiable tendency of most human beings to overconsume. We will again look at the extent and depth of our gluttony and the transformative alternatives, through a physical, mental, emotional, and spiritual lens.

Webster's defines *consumption* as both "a using up of goods and services" and "a wasting away of the body." Although the latter definition tends to refer to diseases that cause this wasting away, such as tuberculosis, it is ironic that our excessive consumption has literally wasted away many individuals' health and potential, in addition to the well-being of our one and only inhabitable planet.

Barbara Kingsolver, one of my favorite novelists and poets and an extraordinary American, recently took up farming and embraced a lifestyle in which she and her family choose to eat locally. She describes her reasons for doing this in her book *Animal, Vegetable, Miracle: A Year of Food Life*:

> If a middle-aged woman studying agriculture seems strange, try this on for bizarre: Most of our populace and all our leaders are participating in a mass hallucinatory fantasy in which the megatons of waste we dump in our rivers and bays are not poisoning the water, the hydrocarbons we pump into the air are not changing the climate, overfishing is not depleting the oceans, fossil fuels will never run out, wars that kill masses of civilians are an appropriate way to keep our hands on what's left, we are not desperately overdrawn at the environmental bank and, really, the kids are all right.

Although her response didn't cover all of the unconscious and unhealthy choices we are making, it did nail the majority of them— those that are of utmost concern for our personal and global health and sustainability and are largely within our individual powers to dramatically change. It is radically transforming and empowering when we fully digest the fact that our moment-to-moment, conscious lifestyle choices pretty much determine whether we prevent and cure our chronic diseases, save money, and help reverse global warming. We can awaken to the power inherent in our lifestyle choices to create win-win choices and consequences, individually and collectively. Welcome to our Ricer family, which has this goal as a daily priority!

Organic Foods, the Best Investment
We Can Make

Most people are unaware that organic foods have consistently and significantly shown greater nutritional content than their conventional counterparts, from a few percent to more than 20 percent for certain minerals and, on average, about 30 percent in the case of antioxidants. These figures are not hopeful wild guesses but were reported by Dr. Charles Benbrook, the chief scientist for the Organic Center, whose January 2008 PowerPoint presentation for the Oregon Tenth's Annual Meeting synthesized eighty-eight peer-reviewed studies that have compared the nutrient content of organic and conventionally grown foods. Dr. Alan Greene, the former chairman of the board for the Organic Center, as well as a teacher at Stanford University School of Medicine, invites you to read the report they sponsored for the American Association for the Advancement of Science, "Still No Free Lunch: Nutrient Levels in U.S. Food Supply Eroded by Pursuit of High Yields" by Brian Halweil. I will share a few highlights here:

- Two British nutritionists, R. A. McCance and E. M. Widdowson, in the middle of the twentieth century suggested that the future of their nation was being threatened by food processing, neglect of manure, and the disappearance of the practice of crop rotation. When these data were reanalyzed, "marked reductions" of seven minerals in twenty fruits and twenty vegetables from the 1930s to the 1980s were found, and the study concluded that "in every sub group of foods investigated there has been a substantial loss in their mineral content."
- Another British analysis found that the potassium content in spinach dropped 53 percent, its iron 60 percent, its phosphorus 70 percent, and its copper 96 percent, and the iron content of meat products declined by an average of 54 percent.
- Another sobering confirmation of these nutritionally inferior changes was published by Donald Davis and his colleagues at the Biochemical Institute at the University of Texas in

Austin, who studied fifty-year changes in U.S. Department of Agriculture food composition data for thirteen nutrients in forty-three commonly consumed fruits and vegetables. Declines in median concentrations of six nutrients from the 1950s to 1999 included a 6 percent decline in protein, a 9 percent decline in phosphorus, a 15 percent decline in iron, a 16 percent decline in calcium, a 20 percent decline in vitamin C, and a 38 percent decline in riboflavin.

- In addition, research from the Department of Agriculture compared the micronutrient content of fourteen different varieties of wheat introduced from 1873 to 2000, a period during which the amount of grain harvested more than tripled per acre. Although during those 130 years, the yield of the common U.S. hard red winter wheat crop soared, its nutritional content declined dramatically: iron by 28 percent, zinc by about 34 percent, and selenium by about 36 percent.

These nutritional reductions are taking a serious toll on our health, with the folks at the top of the food chain in agribusiness and politics being the main financial beneficiaries.

These few examples provide just a small cross-section of the mind-boggling data found in the aptly titled review. While we may think that our producing more food and paying a lower percentage of our income for groceries than ever before are good things, many of the real costs of our food are hidden. These hidden costs, which we as taxpayers finance, are beginning to be noticed by an increasingly larger and sicker population.

While 66 percent of U.S. adults are overweight or obese, approximately 840 million people worldwide suffer from chronic hunger, and more than 3 billion—or half of the world's population—suffer from an insidious deficiency of particular nutrients. Many are unconsciously supporting our conventional farming system, which is focused on making greater profits for agribusiness giants, while narrowing our seed and food choices to those that are more lucrative yet nutritionally inferior. Huge agribusinesses also increase our dependence on chemicals (pesticides, insecticides, and fertilizers), petroleum (a major contributor to global warming), and other costly farm-related products, as well as tragically degrading our natural resources. To counteract this, we have a choice to become conscious and become part of the solution by buying more organic foods.

Genetically Modified Organisms (GMO) = Genetically Engineered (GE)

For generations, farmers have adapted their crops to specific farming conditions and needs. They have selected seeds and created hybrids by cross-breeding plants that occur naturally to protect their crops and encourage their growth. The changes or mutations that helped a species survive were the traits in a species that were then more likely to be passed on to the next generation.

But biotechnology has taken this concept to the lab and has attempted to improve crops, primarily by increasing yields, through a process called genetic engineering, in which genetic material (DNA) is taken from one organism and inserted into the cells of another organism. Genetically modified organisms, or GMOs, could never occur in nature; they are man-made organisms.

First, a carrier or vector is needed to "smuggle" the gene of interest into the target organism. Because organisms are naturally designed to protect their cells from invasion, one might question the intelligence of forcing bacteria and viruses into cells that have evolved to keep them out. Yet we have allowed this, albeit unknowingly, and now the majority of Americans eat GMO foods numerous times a day, as unconscious participants in the largest uncontrolled experiment in the history of the world!

Megan Thompson, the executive director of the Non-GMO Project, recently cited worldwide consumer resistance to GM foods, with thirty-six countries either restricting or banning GMOs because of safety concerns. She also revealed Americans' ignorance of GMOs' prevalence when she shared how 90 percent of consumers say they won't eat GM foods, despite the fact that they had eaten them for breakfast! Today, more than sixty varieties of GM foods have been approved for U.S. food and feed supplies. In 2009, 100 percent of all sugar beets grown in the United States were genetically modified, as well as 90 percent of soybeans, 90 percent of cotton, and 80 percent of corn.

Although this new method of farming was initially sold as a way to increase yields and feed the starving masses, prevent vitamin A blindness in Africa, and reduce our pesticide needs, it has fallen far short of this sales pitch. Furthermore, the spread of genetically engineered (GE) agriculture has made farmers dependent on their more expensive seeds, equipment, and foreign oil and has threatened our biodiversity beyond our worst imaginings. Ninety-seven percent of the varieties of vegetables that were grown by our ancestors are now extinct. This new monoculture causes a greater susceptibility to disease in plants, increasing the need for pesticides and fertilizers, and it results in more waste, less delight in a variety of foods, and, on some level, a hole in our soul.

The Food and Drug Administration (FDA) issued several statements assuring consumers that GM foods were harmless, saying that it was "not aware of any information showing that foods derived by these new methods differ from other foods in any meaningful or uniform way." Author Jeffrey M. Smith presents a different opinion in his book *Genetic Roulette*. In it, he interviewed Dr. Michael Antoniou, a senior lecturer in molecular genetics at the Guy Kings and St. Thomas' School of Medicine in London, who believes that GM foods are inherently different at the cellular level. At a public hearing in London, Dr. Antoniou said, "In marked contrast to sexual reproduction, GM allows the isolation, cutting, joining, and transfer of single or multiple genes between totally unrelated organisms, circumventing natural species barriers. As a result, combinations of genes are produced that would never occur naturally." It is the imprecision in the way that these genes are combined and the unpredictable nature of how these newly introduced genes will react in their new host environments that make them dangerous unless they are regulated.

But isn't the U.S. government responsible for the safety and quality of our food supply? In fact, our foods are regulated by three different government organizations: the FDA, the Environmental Protection Agency (EPA), and the U.S. Department of Agriculture (USDA).

The FDA first established its policy on GMO testing in 1992. The leader of this movement was Dan Quayle, who at that time was the U.S. vice president and the chair of the Council of Competitiveness. Vice President Quayle wanted the United States to be progressive in this new agricultural market, and he didn't want red tape to hinder progress. Accordingly, the food producer would be responsible for ensuring food safety, and voluntary testing was left to the discretion of the manufacturer. The position of deputy commissioner for policy in the FDA was filled from 1991 through 1994 by Michael Taylor, and under his advisement, the general policy for the regulation of GM foods was that they were to fall under the GRAS List, or foods in the U.S. food supply that are *generally recognized as safe*. Interestingly enough, Michael Taylor is a lawyer and had previously been part of Monsanto's senior counsel; he later served as Monsanto's vice president. Because Monsanto is the world's leading producer of GM seeds, there would seem to be a conflict of interest in its former employee being chosen for a government position in the FDA, which was supposed to decide on the safety of GM foods. The number of opportunities for conflict of interest in this saga between mega-agribusiness and the government employees we have entrusted to protect our food supply is beyond sobering. You can learn more about these concerns by viewing the 2004 documentary *The Future of Food*, reading the substantial summary at www.ricediet.com, and consulting the references in the back of the book for more details on the following studies.

A recent Austrian study found that GM corn has a damaging effect on the reproductive system. The research was conducted at the University of Vienna at the request of the Austrian Health Ministry. Professor Jurgen Zentek and colleagues presented their findings to an expert panel convened by the Austrian Agency for Health and Food Safety. Over a period of twenty weeks, mice were fed GM corn (a GM maize hybrid line called NK603 x MON810), along with a control group of mice being fed non-GM corn. It soon became obvious that the fertility of GM corn–fed mice was seriously impaired; they produced fewer offspring than did mice consuming GM-free corn. In multigenerational trials, mice fed GM corn also had fewer offspring in the third and fourth generations, whereas mice fed GM-free corn reproduced more rapidly. The trials also determined that there was a statistically significant decrease in litter weight in the third and fourth generations in the GM-fed group when compared to the control group.

An independent research study published in the peer-reviewed *Archives of Environmental Contamination and Technology* demonstrated that rats that were fed Monsanto's MON863 maize for ninety days showed "signs of toxicity" in the liver and the kidneys.

In another study, mice were fed GM potatoes that had an added bacterial gene to produce an insecticide called Bt-toxin. Scientists analyzed the ileums of their small intestines and found abnormal and damaged cells, as well as proliferative cell growth. In a different study, rats that were fed GM potatoes engineered to produce another insecticide (GNA lectin) also showed proliferative cell growth in the stomach and the intestinal walls. Note that excessive cell proliferation can be a precursor to cancer.

Several farmers have reported that when given the choice, animals avoid feeding from crops that have been genetically engineered. Jeffery Smith introduced us to a farmer named Howard Vlieger, who filled up one side of a sixteen-foot feeding trough with Bt corn and non-GM corn on the other. When Vlieger's cows were let out of the pen to feed, he was shocked to find that they all congregated around the one side of the trough containing non-GM corn. Another farmer in Illinois conducted a similar experiment by planting GM soybeans on one half of his field. He, too, found that geese ate only from the side of the field that had non-GM soybeans.

Although we may not have yet developed our sixth sense, or deeper knowing, to alert us about which foods are GM and which are not, as the animals in these studies apparently have, choosing organic foods can dramatically help us avoid GM foods in our diet. We desperately need traceability to hold agribusiness companies accountable for the irreparable damage that they have caused and will be causing in the future.

Day 24: What You Can Do

There are five very important actions we can take to exercise our responsibility to consume and make available to our families the safest, most nutritious foods:

1. Vote with your food dollars by choosing primarily organic foods, which by law can contain no GM ingredients. If you are eating more organic whole foods, bought from food co-ops and farmers' markets, buying more grains and beans instead of pricier meats and cheeses, and spending less on costly processed foods and snacks and restaurant meals and tips, you will actually save money—especially when you factor in your long-term savings on medical and pharmacy bills and the cost to the environment.

2. Join the Organic Center, www.organic-center.org, a nonprofit organization that will keep you informed, for free, of the latest research findings and concerns about our food supply. And join its Mission Organic 2010 challenge to buy one organic food product out of every ten foods you buy. Of course, if you want to strive for a higher percentage of organic purchases, by all means do so; the higher the percentage of your diet that is organic, the more nutritious and less pesticide laced your intake will be, and the more actively you will renew the earth's health as well.

3. Go to Cornucopia Institute's Web site (www.cornucopia.org) for the latest on organic news and compliance. Its cofounders are among the most ambitious watchdogs for the organic movement, and they will keep you updated on which dairies are actually honoring the organic certification codes.

4. Explore the Organic Consumer's Association (www .organicconsumers.org), which will e-mail you very informative newsletters for free. This is one of the most practical and empowering organic news sources out there.

5. Commit to taking a political stand to educate yourself, your senators, and other political representatives to demand the labeling of GM foods in our food supply.

Tending the Soil

By now, you may be asking yourself how this could be happening, and, furthermore, how could something this important occur without most of us hearing about it? The answer is both simple and complex, and it parallels what we see in our society at large. Our failure to properly cultivate our soil and respect our seeds, roots, and plants are reflective of our leaders' (and unconscious followers') significant shift from making integrity-based decisions that prioritized what was healthiest in the long term to engaging in agribusiness and political maneuverings motivated by greed for money and power.

When you feed your soil with rich compost and plant seeds that are naturally cross-bred for nutrient density and flavor—rather than artificially altered to increase yield and profit, despite their reduced nutrient density and the increased pollution—we all win in many profound ways. My husband and I were first awakened to this realization about fifteen years ago, when we were among the first guests to have the pleasure of staying at Locanda Rosati, an *agriturismo*, an Italian farm-based bed and breakfast. Most of the food served there is grown on the property. The owners, Giampiero Rosati and his sister and brother-in-law, were (and remain) the ultimate hosts and chefs. We felt that we had finally come home.

Although we share the same last name, we are not literally kin, just family in spirit. Giampiero and his family, including their angelic administrator Simone, turned us on to a wide range of culinary adventures. These could really be more accurately described as slow food experiences, where we became enthralled with actually meeting the farmers, olive oil pressers, and winemakers and enjoying their bliss of sharing such heartfelt food. We later met

Carlo Petrini, Giampiero and Luisa's mentor and the founder of Slow Food. We joined the movement and continue to share with others the joy and importance of maintaining unadulterated foods. In *Slow Food Nation: Why Our Food Should Be Good, Clean, and Fair*, Carlo summarizes nicely:

> I am a gastronome. No, not the glutton with no sense of restraint whose enjoyment of food is greater the more plentiful and forbidden it is. No, not the fool who is given to the pleasures of the table and indifferent to how the food got there. I like to know the history of a food and of the place that it comes from; I like to imagine the hands of the people who grew it, transported it, processed it, and cooked it before it was served to me. I do not want the food I consume to deprive others in the world of food. I like traditional farmers, the relationship they have with the earth, and the way they appreciate what is good. The good belongs to everyone; pleasure belongs to everyone, for it is in human nature.

In 1999, Carlo and others also founded Citta Slow, or Slow Town, with the cities of Bra, Orvieto, Positano, and Greve in Chianti as the founding members. Slow Town is an international association that wants to preserve the quality of life through the protection of agricultural production, the environment, and the countryside. The commitment to being a Slow Town includes allowing *no* fast-food restaurants within the city limits and supporting local farmers by having farmer's markets readily available. In November, at the peak of the harvesting season for olive oil, truffles, porcini mushrooms, and new wine, we have conducted tours of the Tuscan and Umbrian regions for Ricers, with base camp at Locanda Rosati. (For information about our next trip, go to www.ricediet.com.) Due to the fact that we rent the entire farm for nine days and have a special relationship with Paolo, their ultimate chef, he prepares our freshly grown, local, organic foods without salt. The morning starts with salt-free Tuscan bread topped with their homegrown raspberry preserves. During the Ricer tours, lunch is sometimes in another town, but we always return for dinner with Paolo and the family, to organic, no-salt-added meals that are awesome. We don't police the Ricers' sodium intake, unless there are patients with medical concerns and questions about eating only very low sodium foods, so the best organic cheeses and olives are also yours to enjoy.

Our last two trips to Orvieto have included a half-day experience with Danilo, the most respected cheese maker in the area, and his son, Francesco, who holds a degree in agriculture. When I asked Francesco whether his father's cheese was organic, he looked deeply into my eyes and said that his father's reputation meant more than any organic certification. (And as we said before, when you really hear the truth, it is hard not to know it!) After petting the sheep and seeing their green-grass-and-barley diet, we rolled up our sleeves to make the best organic pecorino you have ever tasted. It is hard to say whether it is this delicious because of the lack of chemicals and hormones in the sheep's lives, or whether it is due to your falling in love with the twinkle in Danilo's eyes and the picnic setting beside his three-hundred-year-old home. But then you realize it is all of the above! Being that conscious of your consumption and the true source of your pleasures is truly a divine experience.

Another treat for our fall tour with Ricers was a fireside chat with Luisa, a long-time slow food advocate and administrator for the Citta Slow of Orvieto. She told us about much of the history and passion of the Italian-born slow food movement. If you cannot arrange to accompany us on our November tours to their region and hear Luisa and Giampiero speak in person from their hearts, Luisa's following description (translated by Simona Menchinelli, our hostess and friend at Locanda Rosati) on why they moved south from Pisa to her grandfather-in-law's farm to restore it into Locanda Rosati will be the next best thing.

At a certain moment of our lives, Giampiero and I felt the need to live closer to a natural pace of life, closer to the countryside, and we also thought that this needing was actually felt by many.

Locanda Rosati was born for this reason, an old stone farmhouse, with an old cellar dug out of the tufa bedrock, the wood-burning oven where roasts and homemade bread are cooked, surrounded by a spacious garden that changes its colors according to seasons and offers forgotten smells.

The spacious house that we can enjoy with friends and guests, all around the table, in the evening, with a genuine cooking, laughs, and a good coziness are a unique cosmos.

We basically tried to translate in a real way what every man ideally needs: to create a harmony through easy things like a greeting, that with a table covered with food becomes more than a simple welcome. The smell of a sourdough bread, an omelet made with fresh organic eggs, the milk taken every evening at Cesare and Emilio's stable are the fruits of a generous land, and Locanda Rosati offers them to its guests because it couldn't betray its land.

In the years when I was a Slow Food trustee, Giampiero and I consolidated our ideas; we knew that our choices were valuable, so now the work about food as pleasure and quality of life represents the base of our thoughts, like thinking to enhance local produce is important for history and economy but also because if we close our eyes, we can easily recognize a certain produce by its smell and taste; it is in our DNA, and it lets us dream about our childhood. If I close my eyes, through a sensory perception, I can taste bread with strawberries and I can tell you why: my grandfather raised everything in his little vegetable garden; that was his only richness, and strawberries ripened only in May; a few strawberries were precious. My grandfather washed some strawberries for me, he mashed them up with some sugar, and he spread it over a slice of bread. It was a delight, a sweet afternoon snack! So, through a sensory perception we surely make a mental process.

The slow food movement made a cultural revolution over food and economy, food and pleasure, food and environment. The central element is always the man: if he produces and eats by natural rules, he lives well, eats well, and lets the world live well.

The biggest emotion when I was a Slow Food trustee was the meeting with Terra Madre, at Salone del Gusto in Torino, a big earth mother in a big room where farmers brought the seeds of their different lands, and there I understood that the real essence is there, in a seed, where everything comes to life and everything dies.

Becoming conscious of our consumption and distinguishing it from eating with a conventional, unconscious approach involves all of our senses: sight, sound, smell, touch, and finally taste. When Luisa described the smell and taste of the May strawberries her grandfather had given her, I also saw, heard, and was touched by her impressions. I was captured by her words that "through a sensory perception we surely make a mental process." I thought, And also an emotional and a spiritual one. Hearing that her grandfather's garden was "his only richness" then led me to think how bankrupt and poverty-stricken our "conventionally grown" and processed food has become.

Truly being aware and connected to our food includes being conscious of what qualities the food offers. We would all benefit from asking ourselves the following questions before we eat: Is this food grown organically? Why am I eating? Am I physically hungry or numbing an emotional upset with a favorite comfort food? When am I eating? When the food is fresh and in season, or because it is late and I am alone and lonely? Where am I eating? Am I eating locally grown vegetables purchased from a farmer's market friend in a calm, conducive environment or those shipped an average of twenty-five hundred miles with devastating environmental consequences, while I'm being distracted by the TV or sitting in a traffic jam? How am I eating? Am I conscious, mindful, and grateful for all who have grown, harvested, delivered, and prepared the food for me, or am I unconsciously stuffing down the day's frustration, as well as my meal?

Biodynamic Farming Epitomizes
Healing at the Root

The Italian countryside also introduced us to farms that are certified
biodynamic by Demeter International, a nonprofit organization that
certifies farms and produce as biodynamic for consumers. Demeter
plays an analogous role to what the USDA does to certify organic
produce for consumers. The Demeter Certified Biodynamic farming method is devoted to cultivating healthy soil, and thus plants,
and incorporating techniques beyond "planting with the moon" to
produce the best-tasting food I have ever eaten.

In 1924, Rudolph Steiner, an Austrian scientist and philoso-
pher, gave eight lectures in response to observations from farmers
that soils were becoming depleted following the introduction of
chemical fertilizers at the turn of the century. Biodynamic agriculture developed out of these eight lectures given to a group of
farmers. (These lectures, as well as four supplemental lessons,
are published in the book *Spiritual Foundations for the Renewal of
Agriculture*.) The farmers reported their concerns that in addition
to the degraded soil conditions, there was also deterioration in the
health and quality of their crops and livestock. So, biodynamic
agriculture was the first ecological farming system to develop as a
grassroots alternative to chemical-based agriculture.

Biodynamic farming advocates appreciate, on a very deep
level, that soil in its natural state is alive, and this vitality supports and affects the quality and health of the plants that grow
in it. Thus, one of biodynamic farmers' fundamental priorities is
to build up stable humus in their soil through composting. Like
plants, we humans gain our physical strength largely from the process of digesting the food we eat. And the more vital our food, the
more it stimulates our own activity and promotes the health we
desire. Chemical-dependent conventional agriculture has developed shortcuts to producing large quantities by adding soluble
minerals to the soil, much as the average person in the modern
world has turned to fast food for fuel. The plants take up these
chemicals via water and bypass their natural ability to seek and

obtain from the soil what is needed for their health, vitality, and growth.

The result for these conventionally grown plants is deadened soil and artificially stimulated growth, much like the modern human who is primarily consuming empty-calorie foods that are not only excessive in calories (leading to obesity, diabetes, and every other modifiable risk factor of heart disease) but also deficient in essential nutrients (such as antioxidants and polyphenols, which help prevent cancer). We actually are what we eat, and we really should "do unto others as we would have them do unto us." It all comes back!

For the last couple of years, the Ricers' favorite field trips in Durham have been visiting a biodynamic farmer, Rob Bowers, who produces numerous foods that we eat at the program. A self-professed MBA dropout, Rob arrived at his occupation and passion by becoming aware and conscious:

> I have long believed that most of the problems of the world are fundamentally spiritual in nature. That is, the thirst for power, wealth, fame or comfort tends to undermine our ability to see things in a larger context. While technique is essential in applied biodynamics, it is only part of the story. For me, the most compelling aspect of biodynamics lies in its spiritual foundations. I use the word *spiritual* in its broadest sense. Biodynamics demands we untie our finely honed skills of dissection and begin to see and feel things in a vastly larger context. It demands a shift in our consciousness. Not surprisingly, my dance with biodynamics parallels a shift in my own consciousness.
>
> In my early thirties, living the life of a good red-blooded MBA, I began to study tai chi. For the first time in my life, I was able to appreciate the relationship between my mind and my body. I tried to cultivate it further and further. After a few years of focused practice, my teacher told me that the only way I was going to progress was to learn how to meditate. So, I sought out instruction for meditation, and before too long, I found myself taken with formal Zen practice and began to do so at a monastery in the Catskill Mountains of New York.

I was now officially a recovering MBA. While it is folly to try to describe all the effects Zen practice had on my life, certain things stand out. The first was a renewed sense of awe and reverence for life and the importance of living fully and completely. Another was the understanding that how we expend our life energy matters. It is a gift. My teacher was fond of saying, "This is not a dress rehearsal." I knew that the best way for me to expend my life energy, to live with joy and curiosity, was to focus on the essential, that which matters most. For me, that meant growing food.

It was pure grace that in the midst of this revelation, I met my wife, Cheri. In our first conversation, we talked about our dreams of growing fruit biodynamically. Within a year, we were married, had our daughter, Téa, and purchased land in North Carolina. Shortly thereafter, we relocated from California and set out on the task of building our farm and life together.

So what is it exactly that we do on this farm that is different from other farms? The practice of biodynamics can be thought of along two axes, earthly and heavenly. On earth, the farm is regarded as a living entity, and all activities are focused toward sustaining the farm in a manner that creates a balanced vitality. The soil is treated regularly with special preparations that enhance biological activity and fertility. Off-farm inputs (e.g., inputs that are purchased and brought to the farm) are minimized with an eye toward the farm sustaining itself. Compost that is made on the farm is applied regularly in an effort to continually build the quality of the soil. The compost itself is treated with special herbal remedies that enhance nutritive qualities and microbial activity. Crops are sprayed with special natural remedies to enhance metabolic properties and combat disease pressure.

All of the earthly activities are undertaken based on what is happening with the planets, particularly the moon and other close planets. Biodynamic farmers and gardeners believe that the earth is subject to and affected by forces that originate from the heavens. While this initially might raise a few eyebrows, one need only think of the fact that the moon moves over a hundred feet of water twice a day in some parts of the ocean. The location of the earth, sun, and moon in relation to the planets and constellations renders conditions favorable to certain types of activities and plants. The relationships among the planets determine the best times to plant, harvest, make compost, work with the bees, and do virtually any other activity one undertakes on a farm. The result is food that is unsurpassed in its beauty, taste, nutritional content, and vitality.

Steiner believed that one of the problems with the conventional agriculture of his time was that the food it produced lacked the ability to nourish the human spirit beyond basic nutritional content. To get a glimpse of what he was talking about, think of eating a freshly dug carrot out of your own or a friend's garden. Then, think of eating a carrot that was grown with chemicals and then sat on a truck for three thousand miles on the way to your grocery store (the way most in this country get their carrots). Again, it is not a stretch to get a sense for the difference.

Although I have consciously pursued the healthiest food I can find for the last four decades, Rob has taken my appreciation of high-quality food to a new level. Meeting a farmer who plays classical music to his new seedlings in the greenhouse, gets up with his strawberry plants at four thirty on the coldest morning they have known, and lovingly devotes himself to the biodynamic farming method beyond anything I have ever encountered introduced me to a more refined degree of conscious consumption. I highly recommend that you seek a mentor who can get you this excited about producing the best possible quality of food. I'm going out for my second truckload of "super compost" from Rob tomorrow, to enrich my quickly expanding garden plot, now home to eighteen biodynamically grown tomatoes. Who would dare offer them anything but the ultimate nourishment and environment, after seeing the tender loving care these plants have known?

Consciously Constructing a Game Plan

Although few consumers yet realize that buying organic food is one of the worthiest investments they can make for their health and the planet's recovery, the more I learn about our food supply, the more convinced I am that this is so. We now have decades of good research showing marked reductions in minerals, protein, and vitamins in conventionally grown foods. While conventional farming's profit-focused, yield-enhancing methods have created significant declines in the nutritional content of our foods, fortunately organic farmers and researchers have shown that we can learn from our mistakes, reverse these trends, and actually increase the nutrient content of our crops and the health of our soil. In fact, *Science* magazine published an article titled "Soil Quality and Financial Performance of Biodynamic and Conventional Farms in New Zealand," which showed comparisons of sixteen adjacent farms and proved that biodynamic farms not only produced superior soil but were also as financially viable as conventional farms. So it is possible to create better soil, while being financially rewarded and growing healthier food. For the best reader-friendly summary of the organic versus conventional farming research, please visit www.organic-center .org/reportfiles/Yield_Density_Final.pdf.

In the resource section you will find a practical guide on how to buy and eat the best food possible ("Assessing the True Cost of Your Food"), which is based on our program's practices and speaks louder than words; we believe that organic foods are safer and more nutritious and worth the price. Serving the healthiest locally grown, organic food reflects the nutritional and spiritual truths we espouse. How else could we teach with integrity than to walk our talk?

For those who are not yet convinced to buy primarily organic at this time, it is of utmost importance to prioritize buying organic where it matters most. The higher a food is on the food chain, the more toxic and potentially unhealthy that food can be. Prioritize your organic purchases to include meat and dairy and the following fruits and vegetables. The domestically grown fruits and vegetables posing the greatest pesticide risk are cranberries, nectarines, peaches, strawberries, pears, apples, cherries, cantaloupe, green beans, bell peppers, celery, cucumber, potatoes, tomatoes, peas, and lettuce. The imported fruits and vegetables that are usually most contaminated with pesticides include grapes, nectarines, peaches, pears, strawberries, cherries, cantaloupe, apples, bell peppers, lettuce, cucumbers, celery, tomatoes, green beans, broccoli, peas, and carrots. To obtain your own pocket-size, colorful, and complimentary copy, simply order it from www.organic-center .org/reportfiles/TOC_Pocket_Guide.pdf.

The other advantage that organic certification offers is that it is the best guarantee you have that the product does not contain genetically modified foods. Because almost all sugar beets grown in the United States are GM, as well as 90 percent of the soybeans, 90 percent of the cotton, and 80 percent of all corn, it would also be worthwhile to prioritize these as organic purchases. (GM beet sugar might simply be listed as "sugar," so look for organic cane sugar or honey instead.) For example, you may have noticed that your Week 2 menu for Saturday's lunch specifies organic corn chips, which reminds you to buy organic corn products.

Another way to buy more nutritious and usually less chemically laden foods is by buying locally, which often allows you the pleasure of meeting the farmer who grew the food. Like most important and critically needed changes in culturally created problems, the power of the people's voices is changing our food-procurement options and improving our quality of food more than anything our public servants have done. Farmer's markets and food co-ops are becoming very popular and are often able to provide superior nutritional value for less cost. Since 1994, the USDA has published the National Directory of Farmers Markets, which lists all farmer's markets operating in the United States; it is updated every two years. In 1994, the USDA documented 1,755 farmer's markets, and in 2008, there were 4,685. The USDA Web site will lead you to the closest farmer's market in your area (www.ams.usda.gov/ farmersmarkets/). My favorite source is direct from the closest organic farmer; simply go to www.localharvest.org and explore the community-supported agriculture (CSA) and other farmers after typing your address. The closest farmers to you should appear, and many of them will be organic. CSAs are an opportunity to co-op with local farmers; your upfront fees support the farmers, which then entitles you to get a percentage of their harvest, and some even deliver their fresh produce to your door.

Day 25: Assess the True Cost of Your Food

Before your next visit to the farmer's market, food co-op, or chain grocery store, photocopy one of the sample menus from chapter 2 and the grocery list in appendix A and consult "Assessing the True Cost of Your Food" in appendix B. As you shop for the ingredients you need to create the week's recipes, these materials will assist you in becoming more informed on whether your choice is organic and how many miles that food traveled to reach you. Don't hesitate to ask the produce manager the geographical source of the foods you want to buy. It is his or her job to know the products he or sells, even if that means checking the bulk container for the requested information. Before you go shopping, be sure to also bring your copy of the least and most important foods to buy organic (from www.organic-center.org/reportfiles/TOC_Pocket_Guide.pdf). Commit to doing this exercise for one week, but if you do it for a month, that would really be an eye-opener and paradigm shifter!

During our last Rice Diet Program reunion, a couple of carloads of Ricers and I went on a farmer's market treasure hunt, all of us armed with the questions from "Assessing the True Cost of Your Food." This was an enlightening exercise in conscious consumption. Initially, some people felt shy about asking the farmers whether their foods were organic and how far they had commuted that day, but we soon got excited to discover the truth about our projected menu items. We also became aware of how some foods cost more and others less than regular, conventionally grown grocery store items, but that most organic foods were priced higher for good reasons. After you meet a few organic farmers and talk with them about what got them interested in organic farming, how they keep the pests off their tomatoes, why they chose to be certified organic or not, you gain a whole new appreciation for why these foods cost more: organic foods are *worth* more. I firmly believe that either you pay the grocer now or you pay the doctor and pharmacist later.

Awaken to the Myths about Meat

One of our most destructive dietary myths, which many people from developed countries still mindlessly repeat, is the belief that we need to eat meat and animal products to get enough protein. Those with the money to perpetuate these myths will continue to do so as long as you unconsciously choose to believe them and buy their products. With respect to space and having mentioned the research proving the nutritional superiority and adequacy of nutrients in a semivegetarian diet in my previous three books, I will simply summarize by saying this: if you eat primarily whole grains, beans, and fresh, locally grown produce daily, and focus on consuming a lot of dark-green leafy vegetables, you will enjoy the healthiest diet on earth, which will be more profoundly healing for your body and the planet than any other single act you can do! If you want to include some dairy products, especially yogurt, choose the organic brands that honestly follow the organic certification guidelines. Remember that the latest and most accurate recommendations are made by the Cornucopia Institute, at www.cornucopia.org. It is the most respected watchdog for the organic movement and is extremely helpful at keeping us informed about companies that claim to be organic but often are not, such as the Horizon brand.

All Organic Is Not the Same

One of the main issues the Cornucopia Institute tracks has been the corporate takeover of organic agriculture. Nowhere has this been more evident than in the dairy sector. The Horizon label was acquired by the agribusiness behemoth Dean Foods.

(continued)

The $12 billion corporation, based in Dallas, controls about fifty separate milk labels around the country, Horizon being only one of them. Horizon has built a leading market share by producing much of its milk on corporate-controlled industrial dairies, in desertlike conditions in Idaho and New Mexico, managing upward of eight thousand cattle. It has also purchased milk from independent suppliers that milk as many as ten thousand cows in a single facility. The average organic dairy farmer in the United States milks around sixty cows.

After selling its brand to Dean Foods, the original investors in Horizon launched another company, named Aurora Dairy. Aurora specializes in supplying private-label "organic" milk to the nation's leading supermarkets and big-box stores, including Walmart, Costco, Target, and Safeway. Aurora operates five separate "factory farms," managing ten to twenty thousand cows, in Texas and Colorado (the company's own public estimates vary widely).

Cornucopia has filed legal complaints against a number of dairies associated with Dean Foods/Horizon and Aurora. The largest dairy in the country, selling purportedly organic milk, a Horizon supplier, was decertified. The ten-thousand-cow operation in Pixley, California, was a confinement feedlot, and the cattle were not grazed as required by law. According to documents obtained under the Freedom of Information Act, the giant Horizon supplier could not demonstrate that all of its animals were truly qualified to produce organic milk.

In late 2007, after investigating Cornucopia's legal complaint against Aurora Dairy, the USDA found that Aurora had "willfully" violated fourteen aspects of the law, including not grazing its cattle and illegally bringing conventional animals into its operation. The political appointees who ran the USDA at the time overruled career civil servants, who had intended to decertify the $100 million operation, and placed Aurora on a one-year probation.

(continued)

The good news for consumers is that the vast majority of all dairy brands are made by companies of true integrity and with milk from farms that respect the spirit and the letter of the organic law.

As consumers, we have a unique opportunity to vote with our dollars in the marketplace for a different kind of environmental ethic, using more humane animal husbandry practices. And by purchasing organic foods and paying a little bit more by choosing reputable brands, we're ensuring that the hardworking farm families who produce our food are fairly compensated.

The Cornucopia Institute has a comprehensive report on organic dairy foods that is available on its Web site. It includes a scorecard rating the country's approximately 115 organic dairy brands, based on their ethical approach to milk production. In 2009, Cornucopia also released a similar report and scorecard rating organic soy food products. This will help discerning consumers choose organic soy products made from organic American soybeans, which are getting more scarce by the day, rather than food items made from soybeans imported from China.

Since reading *Diet for a Small Planet* by Frances Moore Lappé in 1971, I have become increasingly aware of many dangers in our excessive consumption of animal products. Now, almost four decades later, the hazards of eating animals have grown exponentially. The worst animal husbandry practices include the variety of unnatural, unhealthful, and exploitative agents that are used in the production of meat, such as antibiotics and growth-promoting hormones, and the inherent cruelty of raising animals in unnaturally restrictive environments and forcing them to eat foods they would never naturally choose, given their innate preference for green grass over GM corn.

Safety issues about using growth-promoting hormones in animal production have multiplied over the years. Once again, Europeans have exhibited a more conscious response to agribusiness's and government's relentless pursuit of profit rather than safety and quality. Europeans banned growth hormones in 1988, while the vast majority of U.S. ranchers still utilize them. A joint effort of scientists from the United States and Denmark compiled data through the Study for Future Families, a five-state, multicenter study of pregnancy outcomes from 1999 to 2005. When they examined the effect of a mother's beef consumption on her adult son's reproductive health and capabilities, they found that sons born to frequent beef-consuming mothers (more than seven servings per week) were three times more likely to meet the World Health Organization's criteria for impaired fertility than were sons from moms who ate less beef. Although there is no way to know definitively at this point, the scientists concluded that steroid exposure from conventional beef was the most probable explanation for these remarkable findings.

Besides the dangers of our consuming hormones in meat and their contaminating the environment and the surrounding wildlife, there is also growing concern that links conventional meat-processing techniques to the increased incidence of E. coli in beef. In 2007, twenty-one million pounds of hamburger from Topps were recalled because of E. coli contamination. The January–February 2008 issue of Organic Processing magazine reported that "possible explanations include weather stress, mixing contaminated distillers' grain from ethanol production plants into cattle feed rations, and, most worrisome, a genetic adaptation of the bacteria to become more virulent or resistant to the chemicals used to wash conventional beef carcasses in slaughter plants." Given the wide range of contaminants in conventionally grown foods, it is nearly impossible to determine what caused the E. coli contamination, but it is yet another reason, if you need one, to buy and eat organic foods and less animal products.

A Consciousness Wake-Up Call about Antibiotic Use

Although the use of subtherapeutic levels of antibiotics to prevent animal diseases and promote their growth has been controversial for more than four decades, there is now powerful evidence to bolster the good common sense not to use them. Despite research by the U.S. Centers for Disease Control during 1998–2005 that established clear causal relationships between the use of antibiotics on the farm and the emergence of newly resistant strains of bacteria that then moved into the human population, little has changed on the farm and in the federal regulatory agencies' actions. Now, fifty years after the antibiotics were first fed to broilers to enhance weight gain, the startling results are in from the first study to show a significantly higher presence of antibiotic-resistant bacteria in poultry workers. When poultry workers were compared to people in the same community who did not work on a chicken farm, they were found to have thirty-two times the likelihood of carrying multidrug-resistant *E. coli*! And guess what? This study, just like the previous few hundred, was discounted as providing insufficient evidence to support changes in the use of drugs on farm animals and in public policies that are responsible for our health. The more I learn about these problems with the U.S. food supply, the ineptness of our political system, and the way we treat animals, the more I appreciate the delicious flavors of my organic vegetarian dishes. Note that my three previous books (*Heal Your Heart, The Rice Diet Solution*, and *The Rice Diet Cookbook*) contain more than 450 recipes, and there are numerous others on our Web site, www.ricediet.com.

How Big a Serving of Pesticides and Insecticides Would You Like?

Few people would admit to wanting to eat any amount of pesticides and insecticides, but they simply assume that whoever is in charge of deciding and regulating how much they can safely consume has their best interests at heart. Wrong. That's exactly the unconscious consumer attitude that has allowed our food supply to become as unacceptably unhealthy as it is. The conventional toxicological perspective that "the dose makes the poison" was recently amended in the toxicology arena to include the importance of the timing of the chemical ingestion. In other words, the dose, as well as when and how it is delivered to an organism, greatly influences the potential damage that can be done. Pregnant women and the babies they carry are especially vulnerable. The EPA determined that carcinogens are ten times more potent for babies than for adults and in some cases up to sixty-five times more potent.

Because milk is often a significant part of children's diet, there is increasing concern about the risk of their drinking conventionally produced milk. A conscious consumer would certainly wonder whether milk is indeed a worthy choice after the USDA tested 788 samples of it in 2005 and found, on average, residues from more than 2.5 pesticides per sample. In a 2008 issue of *Organic Processing Magazine*, Dr. Charles Benbrook, chief scientist at the Organic Center, and Dr. Alan Greene, clinical professor of pediatrics at Stanford University School of Medicine and chairman of the Organic Center, wrote that "most worrisome are residues of synthetic pyrethroid insecticides and other developmental toxins in nearly half of the samples of conventional milk." And, as with the previously mentioned antibiotic and bacterial concerns, the pesticide and insecticide problems affect not only our dietary health but also the environment and everything that lives in it. A study published in *Environmental Health Perspectives* examined sixty children of farm workers, ages one to six, and found fourteen different pesticides in their urine, including seven organophosphate insecticides, which are dangerous chemicals that can impair the development of the brain and the nervous system.

That's right, when unconscious consumers buy conventionally grown foods, they are a contributing factor in their children's nervous systems and brains not developing normally. Yes, consuming conventionally grown foods is taking its toll, but with so many toxins and unnatural substances being used, with no labeling or long-term studies to prove their safety, their effects are impossible to identify. The U.S. public is consuming toxic food in an undisclosed experiment, with no formal control group, which is truly a crapshoot. There are indeed consequences to every choice we make, and the more conscious choices we make, the more likely we will be happy and satisfied with what we have participated in creating. Margaret Mead summed it up nicely: "A small group of thoughtful people could change the world. Indeed, it's the only thing that ever has." If everyone reading this bought more organic foods, there would be less acreage contaminated by toxins, less collateral damages, and fewer resulting diseases. This is playing the responsibility game in a big way, and we get to choose *now* as the time to take off our blinders and realize that our health extends beyond our bodies . . . and that we are all connected. This line of reasoning is not radical; it is simple algebra, rooted in the fundamental laws of quantum physics and spirituality. As Coach Foster said, "Read the clues!"

Reducing Your Carbon Footprint: Eat Organic and Less Meat

As we weave our industrialized web of modern agricultural concerns, we learn other appalling facts about what our excessive animal consumption has created. In *Livestock's Long Shadow*, a report from the United Nations Food and Agriculture Organization, a shocking side effect of excessive animal consumption was revealed: global livestock production is creating about one-fifth of all greenhouse gases, which is even more than the amount created by automobiles!

Mark Bittman, the author of *Food Matters: A Guide to Conscious Eating*, translates the environmental damage from our overreliance on eating meat into this analogy: "In terms of energy consumption, serving a typical family-of-four steak dinner is the rough equivalent of driving around in an SUV for three hours while leaving all the lights on at home."

If you aren't dramatically concerned yet, you will be! Globally speaking, livestock is the fastest-growing sector of agriculture; since 1980, the numbers of pigs and poultry have quadrupled and those of cattle, sheep, and goats have doubled! Although Americans are already big meat consumers, eating approximately half a pound of meat per day, the developing world's meat intake is rising fast and has tripled since 1970. Overall global meat consumption is expected to double within the next four decades. Mark Bittman, in *Food Matters*, estimates that "we currently raise 60 billion animals each year for food—ten animals for every human on earth. The projection is that just to sustain current consumption levels (and consumption is increasing, so this is conservative), by 2050 we'll be raising 120 billion animals a year." The good news is that conscious consumers can choose to eat less meat and buy organic, grass-fed animals when they do; it matters.

As we allow our heads and hearts to choose the best food purchases and lifestyles, for us and for future generations, some people may feel certain fearful beliefs and concerns surfacing. For example, thoughts like, Okay, I'll give up my expensive latté habit and reduce my meat and alcohol consumption by half, and I'll bike rather than drive to the market, to better afford the "true cost" of organic, local wholesome foods, but I don't know if I really have the extra time this will take. First, you really have all the time you need to do what you most want to do. Second, reducing the amount of time and energy you spend on elaborate meal preparation may be a good thing.

Conscious Consumption Can Heal and Change Us, à la Rumi

The satisfaction one feels from choosing foods that are truly healthy for oneself, for others, and for the earth is deeply fulfilling. To be "sated" or "satiated" means "to satisfy to the full, or gratify completely." After you read this book, I don't think you can be truly and completely satisfied with inferior foods that are chemically laden and unconsciously gobbled down. To gratefully, thus consciously, eat your food and be aware of its natural, organic essence and appreciative of its benefits to the environment and to all living creatures, including those who planted, harvested, transported, and prepared it for you, epitomizes a truly satiating experience. Consciously enjoying organic, locally grown foods with this depth of gratitude creates a sense of satiety that won't occur in fast-food restaurants or in many opulent, pretentious, and disconnected five-star restaurants.

Becoming intimately aware of and connected to what you eat can change you; take it from Rumi's poem "The Worm's Waking."

The Worm's Waking

This is how a human being can change:
there's a worm addicted to eating grape leaves.

Suddenly, he wakes up, call it grace, whatever, something wakes him, and he's no longer a worm.

He's the entire vineyard, and the orchard too, the fruit, the trunks, a growing wisdom and joy that doesn't need to devour.

Day 26: True Satiation with Rumi

Today's experiential is truly a treat; you will soon experience the immense pleasure and satisfaction of memorizing and reciting Rumi's poem "The Worm's Waking." Recently, my dear friend Victoria Lee, who has written a book titled *The Rumi Secret*, recited this poem from heart—in response to my asking whether she knew a thought-provoking poem on food. What a gift for her to be able to share something so simple, so tantalizing, so hopeful, and, furthermore, so spontaneously! Memorize this poem, and recite it to a friend or a family member today. A special thanks to Victoria Lee and Coleman Barks, a respected translator of Rumi who wrote *The Essential Rumi* and other wonderful books, for bringing these eight-hundred-year-old words of wisdom to so many twenty-first-century soul seekers. From Middle Eastern roots and the language of Persia, Rumi's words bridge any gulf that man has created. Fill your soul and enjoy the satiety that his words and verse exude.

Going Green and Getting Greener: Meal Planning, Food Shopping, and Cooking Tips

The waking worm's growing wisdom and joy that doesn't need to devour are the grace we seek to find in our relationship not only

with food but with everything in our lives. Whether you feel satisfaction from not consuming beef this month—while knowing the
significant benefit this has for your body and for the earth's ozone
layer—or from instantly shifting your perspective to realize you
don't need paper towels, as I did last month, and simply choosing
not to use them anymore, it is fulfilling and satiating! Read the
many ideas described here, and take on the ones you would like to.
Although a few of them may require weeks for you to embrace and
implement, others, such as using a cloth towel rather than a paper
towel, take about two seconds for you to ask yourself, "Now, why
do I need to waste money and trees and further harm the ozone
layer by using paper towels instead of cloth?"

New Approaches to Food

Buy less meat and more fresh produce, whole grains, and
  beans

Create menu plans, recipes, and accompanying grocery lists for
  meals using seasonal produce (see appendix A).

Plan one-container meals that are fast to make, use few
  resources, and are inexpensive (such as soups, cold pasta
  salads, and bean dips).

Cook large batches to create several meals at once, and freeze
  extras to eat later.

Freeze or can newly harvested fruits and vegetables for later use
  and enjoy the seasonal savings.

Make note of meals that your family enjoys so you can prepare
  them again.

Teach your family, especially younger ones, about conscious
  consumption and healthier, greener foods.

Food Shopping Tips

Buy locally grown and organic foods as much as possible.

Frequently shop at nearby farmer's markets.

Join a community-supported agriculture organization.

Visit www.eatlocal.net and take the Eat Local Challenge: for one week commit to spend 10 percent of your grocery budget on local foods grown within a hundred-mile radius of your home; try one new fruit or vegetable each day; preserve food to enjoy later in the year.

Visit www.localharvest.org for an excellent source of practical information on the best farms, CSAs, farmer's markets, grocery stores, food co-ops, and restaurants.

Reduce or preferably eliminate using bottled water; buying a filter or, if using a well, a reverse-osmosis system for your kitchen water will usually pay for itself within a year.

Buy in bulk (preferably from bins) for less packaging waste; avoid single-serving packages that are not recyclable.

Bring your own bags when food shopping and reuse them.

Cooking Tips

Try bamboo cutting boards and utensils.

Use dishes instead of disposable plates and cups; if you must use disposable, use only those that can be recycled.

Cook one big meal, and have enough leftovers to eat three to four times.

Use moderate heat instead of overheating.

Get organized in food preparation to limit your trips to the store and the times you open the refrigerator.

Compost all fruit, vegetable, grain, and bean scraps, coffee grounds, and eggshells.

Food and Educational Ideas for Inspiration and Success

Grow your own garden or tomato, pepper, and herb pots on your patio (see the resources for recommended seed companies).

Throw out junk or processed foods; start fresh with organic, "clean" ingredients.

Join the slow food movement and get involved with local, national, and international opportunities.

Dine at restaurants that are known for serving organic, locally grown cuisine.

Start a Healthy Dinner Club with friends for inspiration and fun.

Advertise at local co-ops or health stores for cooks to assist you a couple of hours per week (at your home or theirs); this will save you money when compared to restaurant and tip costs.

Clean-Up Tips

Use as little water as possible.

Use cotton or bamboo dishcloths instead of paper towels.

Buy biodegradable detergents.

Make and use natural, homemade cleaners.

Day 27: Choosing to Be a Conscious Consumer of Food and Resources

After digesting all of these unsettling facts about our world's food supply and our global health status, as well as finding out how you can respond in an empowering way, based on integrity and conscious consumption, where do you want to direct your focus? Because we are all standing at different starting points, everyone will have a different answer. To recap the highlights and learn how to make other important choices that can improve your health and promote the planet's recovery, read the following bulleted summary to prioritize your healing goals.

- Reduce your consumption of animal products by half or three-quarters, especially beef, and buy only grass-fed, organic meats and dairy.
- Join the "No GMO Challenge" at http://realfoodmedia .com/no-gmo-challenge/.

- Join Slow Food and attend some local events to meet others who are reclaiming their connection with locally grown foods.
- Volunteer with local, organic food consumers in planting neighborhood gardens, organizing fund-raising dinners to enhance community educational efforts, and uniting farmers', restaurateurs', and educators' efforts.
- Research and support activities that help economically underprivileged people become empowered to grow their own food. You may want to assess the work of Bread for the World (www.bread.org), World Vision (www.worldvision.org), Heifer Project (www.heifer.org), Christian Children's Fund (www.childfund.org), Journey to Forever (www.journeytoforever.org), and World Neighbors (www.wn.org).
- Buy the fifteen-minute children's movie *The True Cost of Food*, which would be the ultimate gift for your child's or grandchild's physical education teacher. Or if you don't have children, offer to show the film to a local summer camp or at an outing sponsored by an environmental organization such as the Sierra Club (www.sierraclub.org).
- Again, end your day with a heartfelt journal entry; you may want to reflect on how your consciousness has expanded in relation to your overall consumption of foods and various products. Get honest with yourself about where you are and where you are going in this regard. Who knows? You may be on your way to heading up your community's Going Green project, with a PERT-charted game plan.

You already know that *diet* alone doesn't create the optimal weight and the good health that you want for the long haul. You have likely proved this to yourself through many previous attempts that did not bear the fruits you desired. In fact, you share this history and frustration with millions of people.

As this book goes to press, the United States is spending approximately twice as much as other industrialized nations do on health care. Yet despite an annual expenditure of more than $7,100 per person, we are in overall worse health than people in most other developed nations. How can the most powerful and richest country in the world be faring so poorly, as we nose-dive, seemingly unconscious and out of control, in such important realms as finance, health, and food quality? If we pause for a reflective moment, we intuitively know that our country's recent financial collapse, our obesity and chronic disease epidemics, and the disastrous plunge in the quality of our food, farms, and precious natural resources are really symptomatic of the same sin—gluttony. The more affluent we become and the more excessively we consume, the less satisfying material things and food become, and the less connected and in tune we are with other people, our planet, and its valuable resources—that is, until we change.

7

Amazing, Miraculous, and Extraordinary Healing

I believe that healing and health are a journey, a process, and not a destination. I believe that health is more than a physical state of being or a physical outcome. Health is both an inner and an outer manifestation of your state of integration with your emotional, mental, spiritual, and physical selves. Healing is the journey of recovering those selves to their wholeness.
—Karen Winstead

Congratulations on having the courage, commitment, and tenacity to move beyond dieting to embark on a *dieta*, a way of life that creates and sustains health and healing! As you have already experienced, profound healings can take place when you become aware of the connectedness of your thoughts, feelings, and beliefs and how they contribute to your physical health or disease. Throughout these chapters, you've seen many examples of how we all experience physical manifestations as outward reflections of our internal state of being. At the Rice Diet Program, I have witnessed this truth again and again. And, thankfully, I have also witnessed profound healings.

By now, I am sure that most people are convinced that they feel healthier when they are in touch with their emotional, mental, and spiritual selves. Conversely, they feel out of sorts or unhealthy when they become unbalanced in their natural way of being. I've noticed that people who experience recovery and healing tend to heal when they have a sense of hope, faith, and belief in the outcome that they desire. This holds true even with someone who is suffering from a terminal or a supposedly incurable disease or mental illness. Although it may seem paradoxical to view oneself as healthy no matter what the circumstances, to do so can co-create a state of peace, which in turn can lead to healing, typically on an emotional level. Yet this often results in a physical healing as well.

Healing is an amazing mystery, though. As I write these suggestions and generalizations, I can also think of cases where the opposite was true: numerous people became healed who were not hopeful, faithful, or believers (in whatever modality we were practicing), but they did show up, which exhibits some willingness to change! We can never fully know how individual people will best be healed or whether they will be or the answers to the *why* and *when* questions that follow. We do, however, usually see in healings an active participation of the individuals' will, as they desire and seek the Creative Force of the Universe or the power that exists that is greater than their own.

Although most Rice Diet participants are able to receive dramatic healing with the Rice Diet Program teachings and experientials described thus far, some of our participants, including myself, have also used other exceptional complementary healing methods and venues of spiritual healing and energy medicine. In Donna Eden's classic book *Energy Medicine*, she beautifully simplifies and illuminates this complex and mysterious subject by starting with the wonderful truth that we are a latticework of energy. She also makes the point that it is not a new idea that the subtle energies operate in tandem with the denser, "congealed" energies of the material body. Indeed, numerous cultures have long described "a matrix of subtle energies that support, shape, and animate the physical body, called *qi* or *chi* in China, *prana* in the yoga tradition of India and Tibet, *yesod* in the Jewish kabbalistic tradition, *ki* in Japan, *baraka* by the Sufis, *wakan* by the Lakotas, *orenda* by the Iroquois, *megbe* by the Ituri Pygmies, and the *Holy Spirit* in Christian tradition." Regardless of your culture or faith, the Creative Force of the Universe is omnipresent in most belief systems.

The descriptions and first-person testimonials that follow demonstrate healing methods such as hands-on healing, axiatonal attunement therapy, Hakomi therapy, and healing breath work—all of which have helped many people, including me. Because some of the complementary practices described in this chapter may not be familiar to you, I simply invite you to read them with an open heart and mind, and if you'd like, ask the God of your understanding to quicken your discernment on whether any of these practices might benefit you on your healing journey. As the following associates who are gifted in healing live across the country, I will trust that with your prayerful intentions you can find similarly gifted practitioners near you or seek counsel with my associates in person or via phone consultation. See contact information in the resources.

My Near-Death Experience and the Power of Prayer

Most of the personal stories that I share in this book describe how I healed at the core from a crippling joint disease, by healing my resentment, the underlying root of the painful arthritic disorder. Many diseases that I have personally known and heard about from others had obvious underpinnings or emotional and spiritual roots that needed healing before the diseases' symptoms would resolve. My experience is that this is the case more often than not, and there are many avenues that one can take to unearth these energetic roots and thus bring them to the light to heal.

Ultimately, I credit God with these revelations. As with all other insights and new understandings, it is our responsibility to act on the newly acquired wisdom and truth (or deal with the consequences and create other learning opportunities!). Other times, as with a viral encephalitis–like condition that I have been healed of twice, there may not be an immediate or conscious understanding of what caused it or a deep revelation of why, but it is more of a mystery that makes you ever more dependent and reliant on the power of God and prayer.

I refer to my previous condition as "viral encephalitis–like" because that is what the doctors called it. The doctors never determined what it actually was but only knew that something had crossed my blood-brain barrier and caused my brain to present symptoms similar to viral encephalitis, which meant that I basically checked out for three weeks. This happened twice, five years apart. My husband reported that both times, within hours, I could not talk, recognize anyone, feed myself, or go to the bathroom. I was basically in a vegetative state and smiled a lot. Fortunately for me and my family, during the first viral encephalitis–like episode, my spiritual mentor and dear friend Reverend Tommy Tyson was still alive. Besides being the most unconditionally loving, Jesus-like person I had ever known, he was internationally renowned for his gift of healing. Within a few days of my first hospitalization, the doctors were baffled, and it did not look hopeful from a physical perspective. Tommy went to my hospital bed, prayed over me, and walked out of the room. Bob, my husband, followed him out to the hallway to talk outside of my hearing range. Tommy turned to Bob and confidently claimed, "Fear not; she is coming back fully intact!"

Bob knew that Tommy would not say that to someone unless he knew it to be true. There followed a long few weeks, especially for my husband, my two-year-old son, and my sister-in-law, who is a nurse and generously moved into my hospital room to oversee my critical condition. She later told me how she envisioned her exhalations filling me with renewed life. I believe her intentions,

Tommy's prayers and the many others that were offered for me were pivotal in helping me come back fully intact.

Five years after this episode, my brain experienced a similar but much more serious trial. Within a few days of "checking out" with symptoms like before, I began to have grand mal seizures. They were so severe that they could not be alleviated without totally paralyzing my body and putting me on a respirator to force me to breathe. For those of you without a medical background, let me explain that being put on a respirator has serious potential side effects. In fact, after a patient has been on one for a couple of days, it is quite rare that he or she will recover with the same or a similar IQ. After I spent weeks in the ICU, the medical staff suggested that my husband make arrangements for where he planned to place me; I was told that those on my medical team had run out of hope that I would return. Yet one person who witnessed my healing in the hospital that day remembers what happened—Molly Anne Tyson, the granddaughter of Reverend Tommy Tyson. These are her words.

I received word that Kitty was sick. Deathly sick.

To this day, I do not remember how we were cleared to enter the ICU. I do remember that many others were not. And I do not remember who led us to Kitty's bedside, where she lay like mashed potatoes. I remember that the nurse was not keen on the idea of us being there, but I asked if we could pray for Kitty, and she allowed us to. We put oil on our hands [Jewish healing ritual] and put our hands on Kitty and prayed. To pray is simply to communicate spiritually, and it looks like many different things for many different people. What I believed happened in our spiritual communication that day was that the power of God was activated and realized in and through all of the many people praying in alignment that day with God, with Kitty's mind/will/emotions, and with each other. That day, her body "adjusted" and came into alignment with what was true for Kitty in that moment—that her whole self was to continue living on earth.

The Lord's Prayer invites "God's Kingdom to come, on the earth as it is in heaven." Christians believe this is possible when the life of Christ becomes manifest in and through God's creation. We, as humans, are invited to live into God's redemption by living out the ways of God and the ways of God's kingdom. If God is whole, then the way of God's kingdom is wholeness. The way of God's kingdom is justice for all creation, mercy for all creation, freedom from violent oppression for all creation, healing for all creation. The particularities of how, when, where, and within whom God's kingdom manifests itself belongs to Mystery. However, to receive an invitation suggests that one will be given at least some idea of where to show up, when to show up, and for what reason to show up.

God is Whole. While there is no brokenness with God, God knows brokenness.

Intimately. Through the Person of Jesus, God is in full solidarity with the brokenness of creation. When once all of creation was whole in God, God's creation became fragmented, broken, making its myriad departures from Truth and True Self as time and history testify. When once there was no sickness, disease, violence, and death, there is all of it now, for creation has not yet entered into the fullness of its redemption in and through the risen Christ. Therefore, creation continues to exist in the tension of the "Now" and the "Not Yet." Basic eschatology tells us this. Though creation lives somewhere "Between the Times," the fullness of God has been expressed to and through creation in the Person of Jesus Christ. The possibility for redeeming creation to wholeness is Jesus the Christ—Son of God, Son of Man; the point at which [or rather, the Person in which] divinity and creation become One. This supernatural union—this "return to wholeness," if you will—is the journey into which God's creation is invited. What is more, creation is empowered to live into this invitation through the indwelling of the Spirit of God, or the Holy Spirit.

While those of you who are Christian are likely nodding your heads, dancing around, or breaking out in song, others may feel uncomfortable that Molly Anne has so strongly proclaimed her Christian belief that Jesus is the Son of God and that as part of the Trinity with God and the Holy Spirit, he has the power to move through her and heal others.

Day 28: *Cultivating a Spiritual Practice*

I ask you to meditate and journalize on what Molly Anne's account of my healing brought up for you. All I really know for sure is that I have come very close to death twice, with a disease that Western allopathic medicine could not even diagnose, much less cure, and after three weeks at one of the better hospitals in the United States, the doctors had lost hope for my case. Then, after prayer from two or more believers, I was walking and talking within a few hours! Although medical professionals would call this anecdotal evidence, the events described here are absolutely true. And the good news is that we all get to choose whether to believe in a Higher Power. With the health benefits of having a spiritual practice being so well documented, it is certainly worth reflecting on whether spiritual health is what you desire. If not, seek your Truth. Before you meditate, ask your Creator whose counsel and prayers you should seek. Spending honest, intimate time with the most loving elder in the spiritual tradition of your choice may very well be an integral part of the healing you seek.

Hakomi Therapy

During the last few years, we have also been blessed with the amazing presence of Carolyn Craft, who has become a frequent facilitator of groups at the Rice House. In addition to Carolyn's ministerial training and her experience with Gestalt therapy and nonviolent communication, she is a practitioner of Hakomi experiential psychotherapy, which is a method originated by Dr. Ron Kurtz.

This psychotherapy combines the Eastern traditions of mindfulness and nonviolence with a unique, highly effective Western methodology. *Hakomi* is a Hopi Indian word meaning "How do I stand in relation to all these many realms?" "How am I in the world?" A Hakomi therapist helps people study the organization of their experiences. The body reveals and holds incredible wisdom.

Hakomi therapy is a body-centered, somatic psychotherapy based on very gentle and organic methods. In sessions, the body's structures and habitual patterns become a powerful entrance to unconscious core material, including those hidden beliefs that shape our lives, our relationships, and how we see ourselves in the world. The practice of loving presence and the trustful relationship between client and therapist are central to this therapeutic process.

Utilizing the principles of organicity, Hakomi therapy understands that human beings are self-directed and we each carry great wisdom within us. It is in slowing down our everyday processes that the unconscious reveals what needs to be healed. The therapist closely follows and tracks with the client, rather than having a preconceived agenda. The practice of being present in each moment is key to the healing process. Carolyn has combined all of these experiences and trainings with her natural, easy way of being with people. She is a powerful instrument of the Creator of the Universe to facilitate your healing on a psychological and spiritual level. Hakomi therapy can benefit anyone with any problem, but Carolyn admits that it seems most helpful to those who are open and receptive to their own healing.

Not long ago, I realized I was feeling a little stressed out and thought that the recurring stressful, fear-based dreams that I was having were probably a sign that I needed to attend to them and their underlying source. I was also getting "yoo-hoos" from joint pain in my feet and hands that I had not experienced in many years. When I got comfortable on Carolyn's sofa, she asked me what was coming up for me today and said to simply take a few breaths to *become mindful* (not going into meditation) and *notice* my bodily sensations. I immediately felt a heaviness, or penetrating pressure, which could best be described as a stake in the right front lobe of my brain. This is the position that my neurologist's tests have shown that I have a loci, or an abnormal change in my brain, since a viral encephalitis–like episode five years prior. Although it was not painful, I felt it to be undesirable and wished that it was not there. She went on to ask me numerous questions, such as, "What feelings or thoughts are arising from your noticing this stakelike intrusion in your brain?"

I saw the same memories pop up that had occurred just before the last time my encephalitis condition came on, such as the overwhelming feeling that I couldn't do enough to create the changes I wanted in my world. I couldn't change the fact that my mother was dying a slow, painful, and humiliating death, and I couldn't change a business decision that I realized had been costly, in more ways than one. I felt like all of a sudden I realized that my brain condition had to happen to stop my brain from feeling so overwhelmed, because I could not do enough to change my situation. My brain could not accept that these things were unfolding just as they were intended to do, and that even though I didn't want either of these painful occurrences to happen, much less to continue for so long, they were there to teach me to let go and let God.

I felt as if my brain could not change gears and move beyond the belief that I simply had to try harder. Suddenly, I understood that I needed to move into a spiritual gear of acceptance and grace, and that if I would not do so myself, my omnipotent Creator would unplug my circuitry for a while. It was very interesting that this viral encephalitis–like condition has occurred twice, five years apart, and that this was my five-year anniversary! It almost seemed like at that moment, I was able to understand or catch it before I created a need to relive it again! Toward the end of my session, Carolyn asked again how I felt *in my body*. I'm incapable of describing in words the blissful wave of unconditional love that swept over me, more intense than I had felt in decades; but that is what I enjoyed that day. I also felt the presence of my grandfather, who had died when I was six weeks old; I sensed his prayerful intercession, knowing that he too had always struggled to do more.

Healing at the root of a problem really defies description, because we all have such different physical, mental, emotional, and spiritual pasts and perceptions. But, as Carolyn said that day, by understanding "the history we carry in our 'bones,' we become more awake to our present-day experiences. We are then able to release unconscious beliefs and suffering and let the Greatest Love of all fill our heart, mind and body." So whatever we feel in any given moment becomes a little more intense, which allows us to experience more of our aliveness every day.

I would like to thank Carolyn for her wonderful gift of encouraging us to fully be in this present moment. When you seek and discern the best therapists and facilitators to heal your condition, your experiences and choices will be different from mine. But again and again, my most valuable discoveries have simply occurred after a prayerful request and expecting the best! Personal and professional recommendations are also a good place to start. I pray for discernment to know whether the person I am considering for the position of therapist or healer is God's will, and I always judge that individual by his or her fruits.

Axiatonal Attunement

I am frequently overwhelmed with gratitude for the many people gifted in healing who have come into my life. Karen Winstead is high on that list. When people refer me to practitioners whom they think I would like to meet, and who might be helpful to the many Ricers in our community, I often meet with these healers, talk to them for a while, and, if I'm equally impressed, I go through a session with them. I will never forget my first meeting with Karen at our clinic.

Karen practices axiatonal attunement, which is a method of moving and balancing one's energy. Studies have suggested that illness and disease are actually a disturbance in the energy flow (or in the quantum energy) of the individual and may also be due to a disconnect from the grid. The grid is a subatomic field of quantum energy, which is believed to be our source of connection to God. The energy of the grid is said to be healing energy because it is considered

God energy. Because humans are made up of quantum energy, our energy can connect and exchange with the quantum energy in the grid. Since the grid contributes healing energy, tapping into the grid can offer the potential for healing on many levels. Yet the emotional reactions we experience as negative can block or minimize our flow of energy to and from our connections with the grid. Axiatonal attunement can facilitate our reconnection to the grid and enhance our existing connections with it. Karen also works with chakras, which are energy centers along the spine that begin at the base of the spinal column and move up to the top of the skull. Each chakra is associated with a certain color and is believed to influence or regulate bodily functions and organs near its region of the spine. The chakras help balance our physical, emotional, mental, and spiritual health through their energy.

Many people who desire to undergo axiatonal treatments do so even though there is no active physical disease or illness within their physical bodies. They seek treatments as a means of feeling more connected to their Higher Power, to God, or to whatever sense of power and love they desire. Many of us are already in touch with our physical state of being, yet we are not sure how to integrate it with our emotional, mental, and spiritual states of being, nor do we understand their effect on our health. Karen told me that she has witnessed the most profound healing in people who assume full responsibility for their well-being, physically, emotionally, mentally, and spiritually. All of these aspects go hand in hand. Axiatonal attunement can help facilitate their integration so that a sense of connectedness and healing is available.

When I first met Karen, she asked me to lie down and experience her energy work. I lay down and closed my eyes. Yet even though my eyes were closed, I could see the shadow of her hand over my eye area. She then asked with concern, "What happened to your head?" I explained that I had previously been in a vegetative state, twice, with what they called a viral encephalitis–like condition. The shadow of her hand moved, and then, literally within seconds, she asked, "What happened to your pelvis?" I laughed in amazement at how quickly she had detected the two most significant traumas that had ever occurred to my body, simply by feeling the energy a few inches above me. If that wasn't incredible enough, when I sensed her hands return to my head area, all that I could see was what I now call "a purple show." I told her that I wasn't sure what was happening to me but that the only thing visible with my eyes closed was a full screen of purple. More specifically, it was as if I were being bathed in the color indigo blue. I also felt blissed out, as if I'd been plugged into an electrical outlet of unconditional love! She giggled and explained that I was receiving a healing. Her hands moved away again, and within a few minutes I saw little orange droplets sprinkling into my purple show!

I was astounded but asked whether she knew what it could be. Despite the risk of sounding a bit mental, I described to her what I was seeing and asked whether she had ever heard anyone describe such a visual experience. She laughed and admitted that she had not but said that she assumed it was simply a reflection of what she was doing. She explained that when she moved the excess energy in my brain, I saw a "purple-out" because that is the color of the chakra near my forehead, which reflected the healing that the energetic movement allowed. She was moving the build-up of energy she sensed in my brain to the blocked area that had an inadequate energy flow, where my sacrum and my pelvis had been broken in four places a year earlier, in my snow-skiing collision with an out-of-control snowboarder.

She admitted that she did not know for sure, but she proposed that because the chakra for the pelvis area is orange in color, I saw this orange energy drip into my "purple show" when her hands returned to my forehead area.

At this point, all I was sure of was how limited our understanding of healing really is! I had never been particularly interested in chakras, because they either existed as a reality or not, but this experience certainly erased any doubts and indifference I had on the subject. Although I periodically enjoy this "purple show" healing experience during a good massage, ever since this initial introduction to the chakras' colors and their expression, I have never seen other colors. Seeing colors is not the only sign or confirmation of healing, but as we continue to open our hearts and minds to God's creative energy that courses through us, we will become more sensitive and receptive to various ways of discerning its movement.

Karen shared with me a story about a friend named Indi whom she had treated. Indi's case further opens the definition of what it means to reach for true healing. As Karen explained:

The nature of healing implies that we are in an active state of flux with our health. However, healing can be a passive state, too, a state of acceptance and peace. Although many of my clients have demonstrated this to me on so many levels and in so many ways, I recently experienced a significant reminder of this upon the diagnosis of terminal cancer in my friend Indi, who had transitioned from her physical state into her spirit state just a week before Kitty asked me to contribute to this book.

Throughout Indi's tenure with cancer, she maintained a consistent state of peace and acceptance. I can only recall one time, before her transition, when she seemed in pain for one day. Even then, she seemed peaceful and accepting of her state of being, despite the open tumors on her body that required daily cleaning. She reminded me that her connection with me and with others whom she loved was what mattered most. Her desire for her loved ones to know that she was fine, no matter what she experienced, was, for me, a leap of faith into accepting her state of health as one of perfection, exactly as she manifested it. She had healed herself in the sense that she was at peace.

Initially, I could not accept her condition. I did everything I could to cure her. I treated her with various supplements, convinced her to take prednisone to slow the progression of the cancer, adjusted her diet, and ran energy on her daily, even upon her resistance at times. The treatments I administered seemed to improve her quality of life and extended her time here on this earth plane. However, I also knew that her choice to continue in that state was up to her. About halfway into my experiences with her, I realized that she had already accepted her state of being with grace and ease. It was my turn to do the same. I adjusted my approach, giving only what she would receive, hoping to help her maintain the quality of her life. I began to appreciate her state of being and felt so much gratitude for the lessons she offered me and for the opportunity to be of service to her. I learned about letting go and surrendering to the perfection of the process. I learned how to embrace my new definition of health and healing. I experienced a healing.

The healing that Indi allowed Karen to witness and feel reminds me of the one Carolyn gave me through Hakomi; they both were the gift of acceptance and being at peace with what is. Although many in our society feel driven to do more than is our calling, it often requires merely stopping and feeling our bodies to get in touch with our energy. Thank you, Karen, for teaching us that we can tend to our energy imbalances before we have physical pain, and that healing is not necessarily a cure.

Day 29: Tuning into Our Body and Soul via a Technology Fast

Are you ready to turn off all technology for an entire week? That is the challenge of this experiential tool. We are often imprisoned by our unconscious affliction with busyness and have grown to accept this unhealthy and stressful state as normal. Our technology-driven society has only accelerated this addiction to doing rather than being who we really, truly, and naturally already are and as a result is a setup for disconnecting with ourselves and others. As with our industrialized food supply, it seems that the more quantity (of products and money) we strive to make, the lower the quality and integrity of what we are creating becomes.

This practice might be challenging for you and your family, but I was inspired to try it myself after watching *Oprah*'s "Peter Walsh Stripped Down" episode that aired in January 2010. I modified the rules of this one-week challenge to include the following.

- Turn off all technology (phones, computers, televisions, radios, and video games), before and after school or work and during meals, and tune into yourself and those in your life instead. Spend this time with your family and go for walks, read and discuss books, draw, tell jokes, play board games, and participate in other family activities that you may not have enjoyed in years.
- Prepare whole foods, preferably organic and local ones, with your family members and enjoy breakfast and dinner together. The kitchen historically has been the family's hub for healing and the central location for communicating and connecting. Bring that back to your household.
- Clean and organize your house together, taking on the biggest, communal space as a joint family challenge, then agreeing on basic rules of individual and family ownership of different areas (such as laundry should be picked up off the floor by any child over five). Cleaning can be a workout, so make it fun and challenge one another to pursue their strengths such as gardening, leaf blowing, and so on.
- Make a loving gesture (a hug, a kiss, or a compliment) to express what you love about each family member every day. Create a time, either before bed or dinner, to share something emotionally and spiritually significant; this can be a dream that has bothered you, a prayer or a poem, or sharing the most painful or pleasant memory from your day.

I'm sure you'll find this challenge as rewarding as I did and will want to continue it (to some extent) after the week is up. To continue this on an ongoing basis, follow these simple guidelines, modifying them for your family as needed.

- Technology will remain off before and after work or school and during meals. If you feel that the technology fast has been sufficient in healing your family's addiction to technology, you may choose to allow one hour of technology per day. You will need to determine how you will document this and how your family members will honor the time limit.

- Continue to prepare whole, organic, and local foods together. Strive to enjoy all breakfasts and at least four dinners per week together, if your schedules permit.
- Enjoy weekly check-ins, where family members communicate what's working and what isn't, instead of slipping back into a mode of being too busy to communicate regularly. Choose a night for the check-in, followed by a family movie or other activity that is fun for everyone. Go to www.SpiritualCinema Circle.com for spiritually uplifting family movies.
- Keep up the daily expressions of love to your family members. Explore new avenues for you and your family to spiritually stretch. Imbalances in our body and soul not only affect us, they affect our family unit as well. Having a date night once a month with your significant other and a family activity twice a month allows you to enhance your communication skills and connection needs.

Keep in mind that these are only guidelines and are meant to be flexible to fit the unique needs of different families. If you cannot commit to an entire week, for example, try three or four days. Whatever amount of time you have to give, remember to become conscious of the mind-set and you and your family will reap the benefits.

Breath Therapy

Todd Brazee is anointed with the gift of healing. He graciously shared his observation of how important desire is in receiving one's healing. Although Todd's work as a breath therapist at the Rice Diet Program produced some amazing results for many people, his most memorable facilitation of healing was with my cousin Kimberly. She was the most traumatized and wounded woman I had ever known. For those who are still saying, "Yeah, that healing story was interesting, but I'm not sure there is hope for my desperate health condition," Kim's story is for you. Her early childhood trauma led to diagnoses that included schizophrenia, post-traumatic stress disorder, dissociative disorder, multiple personality disorder, borderline personality disorder, bipolar, alcoholic, and epileptic. Although you cannot fully imagine the extent of her need for healing in this short version of her story, simply hearing a portion of it, from her viewpoint and then from Todd's, will no doubt increase your desire and faith that you, too, can be healed of anything. As Todd said, Kimberly's story illustrates the hope for healing that is available to us all, as Kimberly tells us below.

My story consists of physical, emotional, and spiritual sickness, which paralyzed me in a permanent state of bondage. The seed that started this journey was a childhood trauma. It was ugly, indecent, shameful, and, most of all, my secret. Then five years later, at fourteen years old, another secret happened. All those years of swallowing emotions and disturbing fear came bursting out of me in the form of mental illness. The seed was now a seedling, ready to be transplanted into something bigger. What I did not know was that this journey was going to be long, painful, lonely, and was going to get even worse before it got better.

Childhood and adolescence came and went. Both were awful and not what they should have been. Instead, a new reality came to live in my head that only I knew and could understand. To everyone around me, I was delusional. At the time, my father worked for USAID, an agency of the State Department. His assignments sent the family to Third World nations, so from the time I was almost two, I was living overseas, moving every two to four years to another assignment. Just when I would become close to someone, it was time to move. I had found after a while not to get close, so as to not get hurt so much. Everything in my life was temporary: from the country I lived in, to the house I occupied, the people I knew, the school I attended, except—and it was a big except—my painful memories that would be replayed countless times again.

At age fourteen, I was living in a boarding school because there was no high school in Bangladesh where we lived. It was at Kodaikanal School in India where my secrets began to unravel, at least partially. Just a week before my arrival, I was raped by a servant in my home. So ashamed and afraid, I said nothing to anyone. Starting school not knowing a soul and being left alone in another country without my parents created more fear and anxiety, on top of all the other feelings. The months that followed brought thoughts of suicide and feelings of depression. Finally, the pain was more than I could stand. I was like a balloon with too much air, being stretched past its limit and finally bursting. I chose the chaplain at the school to undress one of the secrets that was haunting me.

My conversation with him was not heart to heart but words he himself had to piece together. To him, I may have appeared as a complete mess, but I was looking for relief. I had missed my periods, which led me to the conclusion that I was pregnant. He met up with the vice principal, and the two of them escorted me into the dispensary. I freaked out! What little trust I had left was gone. I ran and ran. Where to go? I was on a mountaintop, up seventy-five hundred feet. A posse was searching for me everywhere, calling my name. I was caught, controlled, injected with Valium, and placed in isolation for days. I did not speak about my secrets again, nor did I trust anymore. My mother was wired to bring me home, and thus began my journey into the psychiatric world that would not end until I was almost forty years old.

I returned to Bangladesh for evaluation by the embassy doctor. The results were good. I was given a clean bill of health in mind and body. The only conclusion to this whole episode was to return to India. The administrator of the school was not exactly thrilled to see me back, but I was readmitted into the school program.

For a short time, life was normal, but with all good things, they come to a pivotal point: go bad or get better. In my case, I deteriorated rather quickly into a dysfunctional mess. I would take hikes in my head that led me to places that only the devil would go. Once again, suicidal tendencies embraced my mind, and the shadows of mental darkness began to overpower my life. I was placed in lockup once again, medicated, and watched twenty-four hours a day.

The U.S. State Department thought it best that I return to Washington, D.C., and go through an evaluation to see the extent of my problems. After a month of probing into the crevasses of my psyche, it was determined that I would not be cleared to return home to Bangladesh. I would be placed in a residential facility for girls in Pompano Beach, Florida, called Chord.

Chord was a place that catered to girls with difficulties ranging from rebellious teenage behavior to deep issues of neglect and abuse. I would, for awhile, be somewhat normal, and then the dark shadow would rear up its nasty head and I would have a jolting freefall that would cause me to plunge into a state of terror. More evaluations followed, and it was finally determined that I had a form of schizophrenia. The State Department decided to recalibrate my past struggles with the present situation and move me from Florida to a locked facility in Baltimore, Maryland. As for my parents, they were sent on another assignment to Cairo, Egypt.

In Baltimore, the center was run by nuns. Before, I was confined to look at and feel the past, but now I had to look at the potential of the present. Physically, I was confined, but for my mind, I could feel the straitjacket loosen just a little to feel God in the mix. The crashing waves were beginning to come as ripples, and the water was clearer than I had seen it in a very long time. My ups and downs became an occasional visitor, instead of a permanent resident. I made an effort to try to seek God. I believed in Him but had not tasted His grace.

I had finished my junior year, and summer was on the horizon. Sure enough, I was getting on a plane to fly to Cairo, Egypt. The embassy there had a rotating psychiatrist, who could evaluate me to see if I would be able to remain and complete my senior year. I had not experienced freedom in a long time, and just the thought gave me a shot of adrenaline that I needed to keep going. Freedom was not the only thing I resonated about. Fear of failure and the disastrous relationship I had with my parents made me think that these were insurmountable obstacles that I would not only have to face but conquer. As I traveled thousands of miles back across that ocean, as I had done two years earlier, an orchestra of memories filled my head and heart.

On June 3, 1983, at the foot of the sphinx, I graduated high school. I had made it, somehow. Someone got me through it. In the back of my mind, I beckoned the thought, Could it be God?

The next six months passed quickly, like a racing river flowing downstream. My father put in for retirement, and the family moved to Florida. While living at home with Mom and Dad, the prevailing winds of circumstances began to awaken within me. I applied to a college in North Carolina and began my freshman year. My thirst to stay healthy was not enough to sustain my appearance of normalcy. The deep-seated pain could no longer be controlled. In secret, I would perform the ritual of "cutting" to offset the emotional pain. A psychiatrist was added to my schedule list for the next two years.

Florida State University was the next thing on my agenda: finish my last two years in college and receive my four-year degree. My emotional state was acceptable. I decided to attend a church, which gave me a chance to forget myself and focus on God. It brought peace and unexpected hope that I would make it again. To my surprise, God provided me with an umbrella that sheltered me from emotional disaster and provided an amazing amount of love and grace to my heart. I met my future husband at the start of my senior year, and for once, I felt normal, really normal. I graduated from college in 1989 and married a few months later.

However, every now and then I could tell that the dark shadow was still scouring around inside me. Shortly after marriage, I became pregnant with twin girls and then with a boy. As the stress mounted, the walls that kept other things at bay started to get some wear on them. My strength swiftly withered and drooped. With denial in place, my skill of checking in and out of reality was given a name. I did not know who I was or where I was. At this point in my life, the flood gates were open, and the weight of it all caused my circuits to shut down, just like that. The next seven years were a lifetime all their own.

I was thirty years of age, and everyone was wondering if there would be a thirty-one in my future. Death was certainly a possibility on numerous occasions at the decision of my own hand. I not only had to deal with the hell in my head but also had to deal with the axis of psychiatrists who thought they knew everything.

My first diagnosis was schizophrenia. As my behavioral problems began to get acute, the doctors would admit me into psychiatric hospitals and add to the growing list of diagnoses. It started with post-traumatic stress disorder, then dissociative disorder, to multiple personality disorder, to borderline personality disorder, to bipolar, to alcoholic, to epileptic, to . . . you get the picture. With each one came a slew of medications, and then another set to help with the side effects. Somehow, I processed all of them at the same time, yet my outbursts would lead to handcuffs, straitjackets, and psychotropic drugs.

Do you know the saying that when the door closes, God opens a window? My twenties were over, thank God for that, and my thirties awaited me. I was still a disaster, but one thing had changed: hope was on the horizon. My cousin Kitty lived in the same town, and she knew a man named Tommy Tyson. He believed with strong convictions that a person could be healed by God with prayer and faith. At this time, I believed in God, but, and it is a big *but*, God was not big enough to heal me. Tommy had several visits with me, praying and anointing me with oil, but my stubbornness and disbelief took center stage. I think even if God had wanted to heal me at that time, I would not have accepted it because I had practically given up. I was not crying out to God anymore. Tommy did not see any change in me, but deep down inside, he had planted a new kind of seed down in my heart without me knowing it. The window was opening; I was just too blind to see it.

Some time passed, and God in His timing was ready for me to go to the next phase. God was moving slowly within me, and I understood why because I was a very slow learner. Kitty introduced me to another man, Todd [Brazee], who believed strongly in the power of God and His healing desire for each of us. He did this thing he called "breath work." I thought he was the biggest scam artist. I met with him for a couple of hours and told him what I thought of him. Right before I walked out of his office, he asked me to let him try a session of breath work on me and then make an assessment.

Todd was able to release painful memories through my breathing. It was a very simple concept but painful. I couldn't see the window open, but I could feel the draft of some extremely needed fresh air. The more time I spent with Todd, the better I felt. Life, something I had not felt or experienced in such a long time, was returning. *Joy*, a three-letter word, was what I began to cling to and embraced with such force as to never let it out of my grasp. The smiles and hugs from my children accelerated my healing, but my marriage had suffered tremendous damage. The battle I was winning on one front, I was losing on another. This caused a setback, which landed me in the hospital once again. If that was not bad enough, while in the hospital, I received a call from my husband telling me that my father had a heart attack and died. The doctors released me in order for me to fly home and attend his funeral.

Upon my return, Todd became quite concerned and frustrated because the drugs I was prescribed put me in a zombielike state. The breath work could not penetrate through the drugs. I had no thoughts and no feelings. I showed no emotion because I had none. Todd got me off the meds, and I began to wake up from the deep sleep the doctors had put me in. God's healing power was able to flow back into the window, and I was able to take a big, deep breath, a sigh of relief.

Reg, my husband, decided that it would be best to move to Florida, to be closer to his parents. Moving was not the route I wanted to take, but I was not really in a position to argue and win. My breath work with Todd would end, and the future would hang in the balance. My support group and friends that I had made were all going to disappear.

Starting over was something I had done all my life, but with each one, a little piece of me would come up missing. Just as before, moving was not positive in the scheme of things. I felt more alone than I had felt in a long time. I learned the hospitals fast and spent a lot of time in them. Finally, I met up with a psychologist, Dr. Marcia Leder, who knew what she was doing. She was honest, trustworthy, sincere, and tough as nails on me. I also met up with a pastor of a church, Kernie Kostrub, who went the distance for me and did not compromise with his belief. Between the two of them and myself, we rode the most dangerous roller-coaster together, fluctuating up and down for years but making progress along the way. They were both on the same page with me, and I know now that God had put us together for a reason.

Then in 2003, my husband filed for a divorce. It turned my world upside down, but this time God had made some other plans for me. It came down to him requesting full custody of the children. I got down on my knees and cried out to the Lord to take care of my children because I knew a judge just might take them from me. I prayed that whatever was God's will, that it would be so. I finally asked for mercy. I surrendered every part of myself. From that moment on, my life was on a new track that did not include any signs of illness. It wasn't easy, but God came to really live in my heart and has never left. The taste of grace is something I experience every day, and I feel like I am home, not physically, but spiritually with the Holy Spirit, walking hand in hand with the One Who loves me. This journey is not over, but I will remain humble in the presence of my Lord and will be forever grateful for His enduring love and mercy for a sinner like me.

For those of you who have experienced trauma or mental illness or who have close friends or a family member who has, you may have found this true story painfully familiar. As I now read Kimberly's account, it brings me back to my many years of researching the "best" psychiatrists around and dragging Kimberly to yet another who I hoped might be the one to finally free her from her seemingly endless, hellish struggle. Then I also feel overwhelmed with gratitude and wonder for the mystery of wholeness and healing that I believe Kimberly has shown is available to us all. Kimberly's desire, open-heartedness, and belief that God would heal her led to a resurrected life beyond my wildest imaginings. (And our inherited Scots-Irish genes for tenacity did not hurt either!) Although I still wonder why some people have to suffer so much more than others do and why we often seem to need to experience profound pain and brokenness before surrendering to transformations and deep, inner healing, it is an oft-repeated progression in our human nature and life choices. All I know is that I am eternally grateful to have seen a loved one who suffered more than anyone I know align her desire, open-heartedness, and belief that God wants the best for her and to have surrendered and received it. She now has more unconditional love and joy than anyone I know and is a walking testament to those who may still need hope that they, too, may be whole.

You may be wondering, What's this breath therapy stuff? And where can I get some? Once again, my experience is that when you pray (to the God or Creator of your understanding) and ask for what you want, with expectancy and preferably with others who share your good intentions, you will receive. That is how Todd came into my life. His perspective of Kimberly's healing may also be of interest to you:

I've been asked by Kitty to share with you a glimpse into Kimberly's healing session and why the healing technique I used worked in Kimberly's situation. The technique that I use is a combination of visualization, manipulating the respiration (breath work), and energy healing. I believe that the body can heal itself, and that healing can be facilitated with the right means of intervention.

When I first met Kimberly in my office, she was a very broken and angry person, reaching for any hope of healing. Her mental illness was causing her life to crumble in front of her. I could see that her family was barely holding themselves together. They desperately needed an answer.

In the first appointment, I remember Kimberly and her husband sitting across from me, sharing one of the most heart-wrenching stories I'd ever heard. Between breaths of emotion, they shared their story with me, and hours later I was looking at one of the most challenging cases I had ever taken on.

Kimberly had been suffering from PTSD [post-traumatic stress disorder], which manifested with both behavioral and psychological symptoms. The painful memories that Kimberly was experiencing were still vivid in her mind and body. Her mind was reliving those traumatic memories over and over, and her body's nervous system reacted to those past memories as if she had just experienced them. Her experiences were literally trapped within her, causing immense suffering to her body and life.

The breathing techniques that I used in her sessions allowed Kimberly to control her breathing and dissipate and release the painful energetic emotional charge from her body. This occurred when memories of her traumatic past would surface in the sessions, overwhelming her with anxiety and panic. Our breathing is the body's natural means of healing stress and emotional pain. The breath work allows the body to process the emotions, which, in turn, allowed Kimberly to mentally process the events of her trauma and assimilate information that she hadn't been able to before.

When Kimberly would have a mental flashback to one of her traumatic events, that image released a series of reactions. First, the image triggered a negative and violent reaction in her central and autonomic nervous system. This caused her breathing to become labored and restricted. The muscles and organs of her body tightened and reacted in a fight-or-flight response. This gave her mind and body the illusion that she was back in that same situation.

At this point, I helped Kimberly to open her breathing pattern, which freed the negative charge of emotion, which then created a series of positive effects. For example, after a series of sessions, Kimberly could mentally remember the traumatic incident without having any violent emotional reaction to it. Simply said, she was able to think about the post-traumatic images as being in the past, without having the experience of being overtaken by crippling emotions. And thus, the trauma was assimilated by the body and nervous system and no longer threatened her state of well-being. This healing allowed Kimberly to experience liberation and freedom from negative psychological, behavioral, physiological, and emotional issues that in the past would have crippled and debilitated her life.

Our respiration has other purposes than keeping us alive. Our respiration helps our bodies to process and dispel negative emotional pain, rather than having that negative emotional charge held by the muscles and organs of our bodies. Although many of us are taught to intellectualize our pain and bury it, instead of feeling it and processing it, we can change this habit and allow our breath to do what it naturally can do—to give us life.

For many years, Kimberly was living a personal hell that many of us will never have to face. She is an inspiration to us all—that we should never give up. As Todd said, "Through this experience with Kimberly, I got to know one of the most beautiful people on earth. She has a heart of gold that holds a lot of love! Thank you, Kim, for showing me that I can overcome anything if I believe."

Although few of us have experienced the dramatic depths and heights of healing that Kimberly has realized or the extreme near-death hospitalizations that others and I have known, all of us have symptomized emotional pain—whether we were conscious of it or not. Becoming conscious of our thoughts, feelings, spiritual thirst, and resulting physical health or disease responses provides significant clues on this journey through life.

In our society, most of us were not effectively taught how to handle negativity or the painful thoughts and emotions that occur during our life experiences. In fact, the inverse is more often the norm—we've been taught or unconsciously encouraged throughout our lives to suppress or disconnect from our feelings. We're told to "just get over it," "no whining," "buck up," or "stop the drama." Many of us learned from our society to ignore, deny, and intellectualize our feelings, which can often thwart the natural process of healing. Even those of us who have healed from diseases that we know were emotionally rooted and fueled still catch ourselves unintentionally passing these unhealthful messages on to our children, in an ineffective attempt to process through unpleasant feelings faster. But pain and disease are just as much a part of our life's experience as are joy and health. Pain and disease are the body's way of communicating and letting us know that something needs our attention. So rather than judge and discount our pain, whether it be emotional or physical, we can choose to consider it a teacher, a loving instructor pointing us to an alignment of physical, mental, emotional, and spiritual health.

Day 30: Healing with Practitioners of Hakomi, Axiatonal Attunement, and Breath Therapy

Kimberly's ability to heal from the most traumatic childhood I have ever heard of has likely spread hope to all who have read about it. If she can gain access to and receive this unconditionally loving

Creative Source and be so totally healed, you can, too. If this approach calls to you, pray that you find someone gifted with the ability to perform breath therapy on you. Otherwise, realize that many people have received substantial benefits from working with Todd via phone consultations; note his contact information in the resources.

Practitioners of Hakomi, axiatonal attunement, and breath therapy may or may not be located near you. Again, I would begin with a prayer asking for the best person for you to be made available. If you cannot find anyone locally, you don't have to be restricted by geographic location. For those who are interested in a session with Carolyn Craft or Karen Winstead, note their contact information in the resources.

Aerating and Composting for Co-Creating and Sustaining Your Health

Hopefully, you have found the many healing stories in this book as inspirational and revealing as I have. I have personally enjoyed new depths of healing by remembering and writing about these experiences, which inevitably take us closer to knowing who we really are. Reading about physical disease being intertwined with its mental, emotional, and spiritual roots and about such a wide range of healing possibilities invites us to claim our power to prevent disease and really live up to our potential. We don't have to wait to contract a physical disease or have a near-death experience to seek healing. It's a natural desire to seek wholeness, to know and really become our true selves.

There are so many approaches and tools for healing available to us today. You will naturally gravitate to the ones that speak directly to you. Sometimes, you might try a new approach that will not produce the results you seek. Don't lose hope—remember Kimberly! Have faith that you will find a therapy that better suits you. When you embrace the idea that there is no such thing as failure, then your definition of health and what it means to heal will change. Now I choose to perceive experiences that I did not consciously intend to create as learning experiences. I shift from the blame response, which so often traditionally accompanies undesired outcomes, to a question: "What is there to learn from this experience?" Continuing to journalize on this can further help us understand root issues and glean deeper truths.

Keep in mind that true healing starts, and is sustained from, within. It's an inside job. The most profound healing can take place when we delve into the thoughts, feelings, and beliefs that contribute to the disease or the unrest in our lives. Throughout these chapters, you've seen many examples of how we can experience physical manifestations as outward reflections of our internal state of being. At the Rice Diet Program, I have witnessed this truth again and again; and, thankfully, have witnessed many profound and sustainable healings.

Recipes

Banana Barley Bread

3 cups barley flour
4 teaspoons low-sodium baking powder
3 ripe bananas, chopped
½ cup honey
¼ cup molasses
2 tablespoons unsweetened applesauce
6 egg whites, beaten
1 teaspoon grated lemon peel
1½ teaspoons fresh lemon juice
½ cup chopped walnuts, optional
Vegetable oil cooking spray

Preheat the oven to 350 degrees F. Sift together the barley flour and baking powder. In a food processor blend the bananas, honey, molasses, and applesauce. Pour this mixture into a large bowl and fold in the egg whites. Add the lemon peel and lemon juice and mix well. Add the chopped nuts if desired.

Spray two 8¼ × 4½-inch loaf pans with vegetable oil cooking spray and dust with flour. Pour the batter into the prepared pans. Bake for 35 to 40 minutes until a toothpick inserted into the middle comes out clean. Cut each loaf into 13 slices.

Yield: 26 servings (1 slice per serving)

Each serving contains approximately:
Without walnuts: Calories 79 (4% from fat), Protein 2 g, Fat 0.3 g, Carbohydrate 20 g, Cholesterol 0 mg, Sodium 11 mg

Allowances:1 starch + ½ fruit

With walnuts: Calories 104 (14% from fat), Protein 3 g, Fat 1.6 g, Carbohydrate 21 g, Cholesterol 0 mg, Sodium 16 mg

Allowances: 1 starch +½ fruit

Banana Berry Oatmeal Pancakes

¾ cup oats
1½ cups plus 2 tablespoons soy milk
¾ cup whole-wheat flour
¼ cup ground flaxseeds
1½ teaspoons baking powder
¾ teaspoon baking soda
½ teaspoon cinnamon
2 medium cage-free eggs, lightly beaten
1 banana, mashed
2 tablespoons canola oil
1 tablespoon packed brown sugar
½ cup nonfat plain yogurt
Oil or vegetable oil cooking spray

Soak the oats in ¾ cup soy milk for 20 minutes. Meanwhile, whisk together the flour, ground flaxseeds, baking powder, baking soda, and cinnamon in a large bowl. Stir in the eggs, banana, canola oil, brown sugar, the remaining soy milk, and yogurt. Add the oat mixture and stir just until it's combined.

Heat a griddle over medium heat until it's hot, and lightly brush it with oil or use vegetable oil cooking spray. Working in batches, pour ¼ cup batter per pancake onto the griddle and cook it until bubbles appear on the surface and the underside is golden brown, about 1 minute. Flip the pancake with a spatula and cook on the other side, 1 to 2 minutes more. Lightly oil or spray the griddle between batches.

Berry Puree

1 package (16 ounces) frozen blueberries, thawed
2 tablespoons maple syrup

Blend the blueberries and maple syrup in a food processor until the puree is the consistency you desire.

Yield: 6 servings (approximately 3 3-inch pancakes + ⅔ cup blueberry puree per serving)

Each serving contains approximately: Calories 329 (31% from fat), Protein 11 g, Fat 11.4 g, Carbohydrate 35 g, Cholesterol 55 mg, Sodium 228 mg

Allowances: 1 fat + 2 starches + 1 protein + 1 fruit

Banana Breakfast Muffins

2 ripe bananas
1 teaspoon vanilla
1 teaspoon cinnamon
1½ cups oatmeal
½ cup water
1 cup chopped fruit (e.g., pineapple, berries, cherries)
Vegetable oil cooking spray

Preheat the oven to 400 degrees F. Mash the bananas in a medium bowl until smooth. Add the vanilla and cinnamon. Add the oatmeal and water and mix gently. Add the chopped fruit and mix gently.

The texture should be loose but not liquid, and the ingredients should hold together but not be stiff. Add a little more oatmeal if the mixture is too liquid and a little more water if it is too stiff. Spray a 6-muffin tin with vegetable oil cooking spray. Spoon the muffin mixture into the tins and bake for 15 minutes or until browned on top. Turn off the heat and let the muffins sit in the oven for 10 minutes.

The muffins can be refrigerated for 2 to 3 days or kept in the freezer for 2 to 3 months.

Yield: 6 muffins (1 muffin per serving)

Each serving contains approximately: Calories 125 (11% from fat), Protein 3.3 g, Fat 1.5 g, Cholesterol 0 mg, Carbohydrate 22.4 g, Sodium 1.8 mg

Allowances: 1 starch + ¾ fruit

Barley Mushroom Soup

> 2 cups diced onions
> 2 cups diced carrots
> 4 stalks celery, diced
> 5 medium portobello mushrooms, diced
> 2 tablespoons extra-virgin olive oil
> 4 teaspoons minced garlic
> 4 teaspoons dried parsley
> 1½ teaspoons dried thyme
> 1 teaspoon freshly ground black pepper
> 5 quarts no-salt vegetable stock
> 4 cups pearled barley

In a skillet over medium heat, sauté the onions, carrots, celery, and portobellos in olive oil until they're tender. Add the garlic, parsley, thyme, and pepper and cook another minute or two. Transfer the sautéed ingredients to a soup pot. Add the stock and barley. Bring the soup to a boil, reduce the heat, and simmer, partially covered, until the barley is cooked, about 45 minutes to 1 hour.

Yield: 10 servings (6 ounces per serving)

Each serving contains approximately: Calories 230 (14% from fat), Protein 4.8 g, Fat 3.5 g, Carbohydrate 40 g, Cholesterol 0 g, Sodium 27.5 mg

Allowances: 2 starches + 1 vegetable + ¾ fat

Bayou Baked Bourbon Beans

    5 cups dried navy beans
    1 large yellow onion, chopped
    ¾ cup molasses
    2 teaspoons dry mustard or 2 tablespoons no-salt mustard
    ½ cup brown sugar (brown sugar substitute is available for
       diabetics)
    10 whole cloves
    ½ teaspoon freshly ground black pepper
    1 tablespoon minced ginger root, optional
    1 cup bourbon

Preheat the oven to 300 degrees F.

Wash and sort the beans in cold water. Place the chopped onion in the bottom of a 1-gallon pot. Pour the drained beans on top of the onion. Combine the remaining ingredients in a bowl, except for the bourbon. Pour the mixture over the beans and add enough water to cover them. Bake the beans, covered, for 5 hours, stirring hourly and adding water to keep the beans covered. Then stir in the bourbon and bake the beans, uncovered, for 1 hour more.

Yield: 14 servings (1 cup per serving)

Each serving contains approximately: Calories 264 (6% from fat), Protein 12 g, Fat 1.2 g, Carbohydrate 52 g, Cholesterol 0 mg, Sodium 10 mg

Allowances: 2⅓ starches + 1 fruit + 1 vegetable

Berry-Barley Fruited Salad

I like to use ½ cup pitted prunes, ½ cup peaches, ¼ cup pears, and ¼ cup mangoes, but the choice of dried fruits is up to you.

8¼ cups water
1½ cups oat groats
1½ cups pearled barley or hulled barley
1½ cups chopped dried fruit
½ cup sherry
1 tablespoon fresh lemon juice
2 tablespoons toasted sesame or canola oil
3 tablespoons raspberry vinegar
¾ cup minced fresh chives or scallions
2½ teaspoons minced fresh mint leaves (about 15 large leaves)
5 firm ripe red plums, sliced
2 Granny Smith apples, sliced

Put the oat groats and 4 cups water in a pot, cover, and bring to a boil. Reduce the heat and simmer the groats for 1 hour or more until tender, adding more water if needed. Wash the barley until the water runs clear. Add the barley to the remaining 4¼ cups water in another pot and bring to a boil. Reduce the heat and simmer for 30 minutes for pearled barley or 45 minutes for hulled barley.

Put the dried fruit in a bowl with the sherry. Cover and marinate from 15 minutes to overnight in the refrigerator, whichever is convenient.

Combine the cooked grains and marinated dried fruit and stir in the lemon juice, oil, vinegar, chives, and mint leaves, but not the fresh fruit. Cover the mixture and chill. Add the fresh fruit just before serving. The grain mixture will keep in the refrigerator for a week or more, and the mixture of fresh fruit can simply be added when desired.

Yield: 15 cups (½ cup per serving)

Each serving contains approximately: Calories 128 (14% from fat), Protein 2 g, Fat 2 g, Carbohydrate 17 g, Cholesterol 0 mg, Sodium 5 mg

Allowances: 1 starch + ½ fruit + ½ fat

Black Bean Burger with Fresh Salsa

Panko is a type of bread crumb used in Asian cuisine. It can be found in Asian markets and health food stores.

6 cups cooked black beans
1 red bell pepper, seeded and diced
1 green bell pepper, seeded and diced
½ large onion, diced
1 tablespoon minced fresh garlic
2 teaspoons cumin
1 tablespoon extra-virgin olive oil
2 tablespoons chopped fresh cilantro
1½ cups panko bread crumbs

Divide the beans into two equal portions and puree 3 cups of them.

In a hot skillet, sauté the peppers, onion, garlic, and 1 teaspoon cumin in olive oil.

In a large bowl, mix the whole beans, sautéed vegetables, pureed beans, remaining cumin, and cilantro. Add the panko bread crumbs and form the mixture into patties. Then cook the burgers, either pan fry over medium-high heat or bake in a preheated oven at 400 degrees F. Cook the patties about 10 minutes per side, turning when the desired texture is achieved.

Fresh Salsa
½ red onion
½ red bell pepper
½ green bell pepper
1 tomato
1 teaspoon minced fresh garlic
1 tablespoon fresh cilantro
1 tablespoon lemon juice
Juice of 1 lime
1 tablespoon honey
1 tablespoon extra-virgin olive oil
Lettuce

Puree all of the ingredients except the lettuce in a food processor or a blender to the desired consistency. Top the burger with salsa and place it on a bed of lettuce.

Yield for the burgers: 6 servings (1 6-ounce patty per serving)

Yield for the salsa: 6 servings (⅓ cup per serving)

Each serving contains approximately: Calories 368 (14% from fat), Protein 18.4 g, Fat 5.9 g, Carbohydrate 47.6 g, Cholesterol 0 mg, Sodium 29.2 mg

Allowances: 1 fat + 3 starches + 1½ proteins + ½ vegetable

Barley and Black-Eyed Pea Salad

½ cup chopped onion
2 cups cold, cooked barley, fluffed with a fork
2 cups cooked black-eyed peas
½ cup diced red and orange sweet peppers
1 cup corn kernels, fresh or frozen
¼ cup chopped Italian flat-leaf parsley
2 tablespoons extra-virgin olive oil
4 tablespoons balsamic vinegar
3 tablespoons lime juice
5 tablespoons toasted sesame seeds

Place the onion in a small bowl filled with cold water for a few minutes, then drain. Mix all of the ingredients together in a separate bowl and chill, covered, overnight in the refrigerator.

Yield: 6 servings (1 cup per serving)

Each serving contains approximately: Calories 226 (28% from fat), Fat 7 g, Protein 7 g, Carbohydrate 35 g, Cholesterol 0 mg, Sodium 14 mg

Allowances: 1¼ fats + 2 starches + ½ vegetable

Braised Bok Choy

1 tablespoon olive oil
1 large leek, diced (about 1 cup)
1 small yellow onion, diced (about 1 cup)
1 tablespoon frésh basil (or 2 teaspoons dried)
3 tablespoons no-salt tomato puree

1 teaspoon freshly ground black pepper
1 large bok choy, diced (about 8½ cups)
1 can apple juice (5.5 ounces)
1½ cups vegetable stock or water

In a large saucepan, heat the olive oil over medium-high heat. Add the leek, onions, basil, tomato puree, and black pepper and let simmer for 5 minutes. Then add the bok choy, apple juice, and stock or water, and bring to a boil, stirring often for 5 minutes. Reduce the heat and let simmer for 15 more minutes. Remove from the heat and serve.

Yield: 6½ cups, 5 servings (approximately 1⅓ cups per serving)

Each serving contains approximately: Calories 82 (34% from fat), Protein 2.6 g, Fat 3.1 g, Carbohydrate 10.4 g, Cholesterol 0 mg, Sodium 87.6 mg

Allowances: 3 vegetables

Cassandra's Carrot Ginger Soup

2 pounds carrots
1 large onion, diced
3 stalks celery, chopped
1 quart no-salt vegetable stock
2 tablespoons fresh peeled and chopped ginger root
3 tablespoons honey
1 teaspoon extra-virgin olive oil
6 ounces orange juice
Few sprigs of fresh parsley (optional)

In a saucepan with a little water, boil the carrots until they're soft and set them aside. Add the olive oil to a hot skillet and sauté the onion and celery until they're tender. Add the cooked carrots and the ginger root and continue to cook for approximately 10 more minutes. Put the vegetable stock, the carrot mixture, and all of the remaining ingredients except the parsley into a soup pot.

Simmer everything for 15 minutes. Remove the pot from the heat, place the vegetables in a food processor, and blend to a smooth consistency. Serve the soup hot. Garnish with fresh parsley, if desired.

Yield: 6 servings (9 ounces per serving)

Each serving contains approximately: Calories 122 (11% from fat), Protein 1.7 g, Fat 1.5 g, Carbohydrate 21.6 g, Cholesterol 0 mg, Sodium 121 mg

Allowances: 3 vegetables + ¾ fruit

Citrus-Kissed Quinoa

  1 cup quinoa
  1 tablespoon extra-virgin olive oil
  1 tablespoon grated lemon zest (preferably organic)
  1 cup water
  1 cup orange juice
  ¼ cup chopped dried apricots

Rinse the quinoa until the water runs clear. Heat the olive oil over medium heat in a large saucepan. Add the rinsed quinoa and lemon zest. Sauté them until the quinoa is lightly browned. Add the water, orange juice, and apricots. Bring everything to a boil. Reduce the heat and simmer the mixture until all of the liquid is absorbed, about 15 minutes.

Yield: 6 servings (½ cup per serving)

Each serving contains approximately: Calories 145 (19% from fat), Protein 4.7 g, Fat 3 g, Carbohydrate 25.1 g, Cholesterol 0 mg, Sodium 3.9 mg
Allowances: ½ fat + 1 starch + ¾ fruit

Dr. Rosati's Pasta con Sarde

  1 pound pasta (linguine or penne), fresh or dried
  4 tablespoons extra-virgin olive oil, divided

1 cup plain bread crumbs
8 cloves garlic, thinly sliced
Coarsely ground black pepper
2 4-ounce tins no-salt sardines, drained
1 teaspoon crushed red pepper flakes
½ cup flat-leaf parsley, chopped

Cook the pasta according to the package directions.

Add 2 tablespoons of the olive oil to a sauté pan over medium heat. Add the bread crumbs and stir until they begin to brown. Add the garlic and sauté, stirring, for about 1 minute. Add the pepper and the remaining olive oil. Add the sardines and red pepper flakes and sauté for 2 to 3 minutes. Add the cooked pasta and toss everything. Add the chopped parsley and toss again. Adjust the seasonings, if necessary, and serve.

Yield: 8 servings (approximately 1 cup plus 2 tablespoons per serving)

Each serving contains approximately: Calories 313 (26% from fat), Protein 7 g, Fat 9 g, Carbohydrate 51 g, Cholesterol 9 mg, Sodium 30 mg

Allowances: 2 starches + 2 fats + 1 protein

Honey Mustard Sauce

As this recipe is enjoyed on many different dishes, you may make larger or smaller amounts as you desire.

4 tablespoons no-salt stone-ground mustard
1 tablespoon no-fat/no-salt Dijon mustard
½ tablespoon honey
½ tablespoon or more dill (dried or fresh)
3 tablespoons water, or more as needed

Mix all of the ingredients together in a medium bowl. Cover and refrigerate until needed. The sauce will keep in the refrigerator for a couple of weeks.

Yield: ½ cup (8 servings)

Each serving contains approximately: Calories 15 (36% from fat), Protein 0.6 g, Fat 0.6 g, Carbohydrate 2 g, Cholesterol 0 mg, Sodium 2.5 mg

Allowances: 0

Hummus in a Hurry

You can order the Marco Polo Hot Ajvar Red Pepper and Eggplant Spread at www.ricediet.com.

>   1 can (15 ounces) no-salt garbanzo beans
>   ⅓ cup Marco Polo Hot Ajvar Red Pepper and Eggplant Spread
>   1 tablespoon tahini
>   1 teaspoon lemon juice

Drain the garbanzo beans and reserve the liquid. Place the beans in a food processor or a blender and puree until they're a smooth consistency. Add the ajvar, tahini, and lemon juice and puree until the ingredients are combined. Add the bean liquid until the desired consistency is achieved.

Yield: 1¾ cups, 2 servings (¾ cup + 2 tablespoons per serving)

Each serving contains approximately: Calories 280 (21% from fat), Protein 12 g, Fat 6.5 g, Carbohydrate 40 g, Cholesterol 0 mg, Sodium 50 mg

Allowances: 3 starches + 1 fat

Jicama, Radish, and Cucumber Salad with Brown Rice Vinegar Dressing

Mirin is a rice wine used in many authentic Japanese dishes. Avoid purchasing Shio Mirin, which has added salt.

>   4 cups medium-diced cucumber (preferably seedless)
>   4 cups jicama, cut into ¼" matchsticks

2 cups thinly sliced radish
1 tablespoon diced mint
1 tablespoon diced Italian parsley
1 tablespoon diced cilantro
⅓ cup mirin
¼ cup lemon juice (preferably fresh squeezed)
⅓ cup brown rice vinegar

Combine the cucumber, jicama, radish, mint, parsley, and cilantro in a large bowl. Toss the ingredients lightly to combine them. Whisk the mirin, lemon juice, and brown rice vinegar in a small bowl. Pour the dressing over the vegetables and toss lightly.

Yield: 10 servings (1 cup per serving)

Each serving contains approximately: Calories 35 (0% from fat), Protein 1 g, Fat 0 g, Carbohydrate 7 g, Cholesterol 0 g, Sodium 11 mg

Allowances: 1 vegetable

Kasha Varnishkes

1 teaspoon extra-virgin olive oil
1½ large onions, sliced into rounds
½ cup chopped celery
6 ounces bow-tie noodles
1 medium egg white
½ cup medium or coarse kasha (buckwheat groats)
1 cup water or no-salt vegetable stock
Freshly ground pepper
½ cup fresh chopped sorrel or parsley (optional)

Heat the olive oil over medium heat in a medium-size pan. Add the onions and celery and sauté until the onions are golden, approximately 8 minutes. Remove the vegetables from the heat and put them onto a plate.

Bring a large pot of water to a boil. Cook the bow-tie pasta until it's al dente (follow the cooking directions on the package). Drain it and set aside.

Beat the egg white in a small bowl. Add the kasha, stirring until all of the grains are coated with the egg white. Fry the kasha in a pan over medium heat, stirring until the egg has dried on the kasha and the kernels are brown and separate.

Add the water or stock and the pepper to the kasha and bring to a boil. Add the onions and celery, cover the pot tightly, and cook on low heat, steaming the kasha for approximately 10 minutes. Check that the kernels are tender and the liquid has been absorbed. If not, re-cover the pot and continue steaming the kasha for 3 to 5 minutes.

Combine the kasha and onions with the pasta. Add additional pepper to taste. Garnish the dish with the sorrel or parsley, if desired.

Yield: 7½ cups, 6 servings (1¼ cups per serving)

Each serving contains approximately: Calories 166 (10% from fat), Protein 6 g, Fat 1.8 g, Carbohydrate 30.6 g, Cholesterol 0 mg, Sodium 74 mg

Allowances: 2 starches + ½ vegetable

Mashed Cauliflower

1 head garlic
1 medium head cauliflower
2 tablespoons extra-virgin olive oil
⅛ teaspoon smoked paprika
A few tablespoons water

Preheat the oven to 400 degrees F. With a sharp knife cut approximately ¼ inch off the small end of the garlic head, just enough to slightly open each garlic clove. (This is done so that after the bulb is cooked it can simply be mashed to release the roasted garlic paste.) Coat your palm with a little olive oil to rub on the garlic head, then place it in the oven on a baking sheet and roast it for 45 minutes.

Cut the cauliflower into florets and put them in a medium saucepan with 1 to 2 inches of water. Boil the cauliflower until it's tender, about 10 minutes. Drain it and place it in a blender or a food processor.

When the garlic head has roasted, remove it from the oven, let it cool, then pop out the cloves. Add the garlic cloves, olive oil, paprika, and water, 1 tablespoon at a time, to a blender or a food processor and puree until the mixture reaches a smooth consistency similar to mashed potatoes.

Yield: 4 servings (¾ cup per serving)

Each serving contains approximately: Calories 64 (4% from fat), Protein 3 g, Fat 2.5 g, Carbohydrate 5.9 g, Cholesterol 0 mg, Sodium 39 mg

Allowances: ½ fat + 1½ vegetables

Nancy's Ambrosia

½ cup cream of wheat, cooked
½ cup canned pears
2 teaspoons vanilla extract
2 teaspoons cinnamon, divided
½ cup oatmeal, raw
1 tablespoon honey
2 oranges, seeded and sectioned
1 cup pineapple, cubed
1 cup grapes
1 Red Delicious apple, cored and diced
1 cup strawberries, tops removed and sliced

Preheat the oven to 450 degrees. In a blender or a food processor, puree the cream of wheat, pears, 1 teaspoon vanilla extract, and 1 teaspoon cinnamon and refrigerate, covered, for at least 30 minutes. Combine the oatmeal, honey, remaining teaspoon vanilla extract, and remaining teaspoon cinnamon in a small baking pan and toast in the oven for 12 to 14 minutes.

Plate the fresh fruit, pour on the puree, and sprinkle the toasted oats on top.

Yield: 6 servings (approximately 1 cup fruit, ⅙ of the puree, and ⅙ of the toasted oats)

Each serving contains approximately: Calories 140 (6% from fat), Protein 2 g, Fat 1 g, Carbohydrate 34 g, Cholesterol 0 mg, Sodium 15 mg

Allowances: 1½ fruits + ½ starch

Nancy's Baked Eggplant

1 red bell pepper, seeded and chopped
1 cup chopped red onion
1 clove garlic, chopped
1 tablespoon fresh basil
1 teaspoon oregano
1 teaspoon paprika
½ cup uncooked grits
2 teaspoons extra-virgin olive oil
1 large eggplant, cut into 4 slices lengthwise
1 whole tomato, pureed

Preheat the oven to 400 degrees F. Puree the bell pepper, onion, and garlic, along with the basil, oregano, and paprika, in a blender or a food processor, adding a little water if needed. Cook the grits according to the package directions. Mix the grits with the puree to make a batter and set it aside. Coat a cookie sheet with the olive oil. Dip the eggplant slices in the batter, place them on the cookie sheet, and bake for 50 minutes or until they're browned. Pour the tomato puree equally over the 4 slices of eggplant.

Yield: 2 servings (2 slices per serving)

Each serving contains approximately: Calories 258 (20% from fat), Protein 6.2 g, Fat 5.6 g, Carbohydrate 42.8 g, Cholesterol 0 mg, Sodium 11.1 mg

Allowances: 1¾ starches + 3 vegetables + 1 fat

Nancy's Carrot Muffins

3 medium ripe bananas
½ teaspoon vanilla

    1 teaspoon cinnamon
    ½ teaspoon nutmeg
    ½ teaspoon ground cloves
    1½ cups regular rolled oats
    ½ cup shredded carrots
    1½ cups water
    ¼ cup raisins (or ½ cup raisins if not using dried cranberries)
    ¼ cup dried cranberries
    Vegetable oil cooking spray

Preheat the oven to 400 degrees F. Gently mash the bananas in a medium bowl until they are a smooth consistency. Add the vanilla, cinnamon, nutmeg, and cloves. Add the oats, carrots, and water and mix gently. Mix in the raisins and/or dried cranberries. The texture should be loose but not liquid, with the ingredients holding together but not stiff. (If the mixture is too stiff, add a few drops more of water. If it's too loose, add more oats.) Spray a nonstick muffin pan with vegetable oil cooking spray and spoon the batter into the muffin cups. Bake the muffins for 15 minutes or until they're lightly browned on top. Turn off the heat and keep the muffins in the oven for an additional 10 minutes. The muffins may be refrigerated for 2 to 3 days or frozen for 2 to 3 months.

Yield: 12 servings (1 muffin per serving)

Each serving contains approximately: Calories 89 (9% from fat), Protein 1.9 g, Fat 0.9 g, Carbohydrate 17.3 g, Cholesterol 0 mg, Sodium 3.6 mg

Allowances: ½ starch + ¾ fruit

Napa Slaw with Honey Mustard Sauce

    6 cups thinly sliced Napa cabbage
    1 cup grated carrots
    ½ cup daikon grated radish
    ½ cup raisins
    ¼ cup plus 2 tablespoons Honey Mustard Sauce (page 258)

Core the cabbage and discard any brown or limp leaves. Shred the cabbage using a serrated knife. Mix the cabbage, grated carrots, and radish. Add the raisins. Toss everything with the Honey Mustard Sauce and refrigerate until ready to serve.

Yield: 6 servings (1 cup per serving)

Each serving contains approximately: Calories 85 (0% from fat), Protein 2 g, Fat 0 g, Carbohydrate 20 g, Cholesterol 0 mg, Sodium 30 mg

Allowances: 2 vegetables + ½ fruit

Refried Beans and Salsa with Chips

> 1 can (16 ounces) no-salt Bearitos refried beans
> 6 ounces store-bought no-salt-added salsa
> Juice of 1 lime
> 2 tablespoons chopped fresh cilantro
> 1 jalapeño, seeded and minced
> 6–8 baked, no-salt corn chips

Mix the refried beans with the salsa. Blend in the lime juice, cilantro, and jalapeño to taste. (Beware of pickled jalapeños, which are loaded with sodium.) Serve the beans with baked, no-salt corn chips.

Yield: 5 servings (approximately ⅔ cup of dip per serving)

Each serving contains approximately: Calories 188 (14% from fat), Protein 7 g, Fat 3 g, Carbohydrate 35 g, Cholesterol 0 mg, Sodium 32 mg

Allowances: 2 starches + 1 vegetable

Rice House Fried Fish

> 4 5-ounce halibut fillets
> 4 tablespoons Honey Mustard Sauce (page 258)
> 2 cups shredded wheat

Preheat the oven to 375 degrees F. Place the fish fillets on a cutting board. Brush the fish with the Honey Mustard Sauce until the fillets are evenly coated. Crush the shredded wheat. Spread the crushed shredded wheat on the bottom of a large baking pan. Place the fish fillets on top of the shredded wheat and press firmly to coat each side. Place the fish fillets on a nonstick baking pan. Bake the fillets until they're firm, approximately 15 minutes.

Yield: 4 servings (1 fish filet per serving)

Each serving contains approximately: Calories 256 (14% from fat), Protein 32.6 g, Fat 4 g, Carbohydrate 20 g, Cholesterol 45.3 mg, Sodium 79 mg

Allowances: 4 proteins + ½ starch

Rice House Mushroom Stuffing

4 whole-wheat salt-free pitas (preferably Toufayan Brand Salt Free pitas)
4 cups coarsely chopped mushrooms (any kind but shiitake)
¼ cup chopped red pepper
¼ cup chopped green pepper
¼ cup chopped yellow pepper
1 cup chopped celery
1 cup chopped onion
4 Toufayan Brand Salt Free pitas, coarsely chopped (call 800-EAT-PITA to order)
2 tablespoons extra-virgin olive oil
2 tablespoons minced garlic
1 tablespoon paprika
½ teaspoon thyme
½ teaspoon freshly ground black pepper

Preheat the oven to 350 degrees F. Add the chopped vegetables and the pitas to a large bowl. Add the olive oil, garlic, herbs, and pepper and toss well. Transfer the mixture to a lightly greased cookie sheet or a large deep baking dish. Cover it with aluminum foil, and bake it for 1 hour, depending on how crispy you prefer your stuffing. For extra-crispy stuffing, remove the foil for the last 15 minutes of baking (watch carefully so that you do not burn the stuffing).

Yield: 7 servings (1 cup per serving)

Each serving contains approximately: Calories 116 (32% from fat), Protein 3 g, Fat 4.1 g, Carbohydrate 14.2 g, Sodium 19 mg

Allowances: ¾ fat + ½ starch + 2 vegetables

Roasted Red Pepper Bisque

1 large yellow bell pepper
6 large red bell peppers
1 teaspoon olive oil
2 shallots, diced
1 large onion, diced
2 carrots, roughly chopped
1 teaspoon minced garlic
1 quart no-salt vegetable stock
1 teaspoon dried basil
2 teaspoons lemon juice
1 teaspoon freshly ground black pepper
½ to 1 teaspoon red pepper flakes (optional)
1 tablespoon honey
⅛ cup chopped fresh basil
⅛ cup chopped fresh parsley

Preheat the oven to 400 degrees F. Roast the peppers in the oven until they are charred. Remove them from the oven and place them in a bowl. Wrap them with foil or put them in a paper bag for 15 minutes to let them sweat. In a hot skillet, add the oil, shallots, onion, and carrots and sauté them until they're tender. Add the garlic and set the vegetables aside.

Peel the peppers (the skin should slide off). Remove the seeds and pith. Add the peppers to a soup pot, along with the onion and carrot mixture. Pour in the vegetable stock, bring to a simmer, and cook for 15 minutes. Then place all of the ingredients, except for the fresh basil and parsley, in a food processor or a blender and puree them until they're smooth. Top the soup with the fresh herbs. This soup can be served hot or cold, and it freezes well.

Yield: 6 servings (1 cup per serving)

Each serving contains approximately: Calories 90 (10% from fat), Protein 2 g, Fat 1 g, Carbohydrate 18 g, Cholesterol 0 mg, Sodium 25 mg

Allowances: 3½ vegetables

Spaghetti Squash with Honey Mustard Sauce

> 2 spaghetti squash, halved and seeded
> ⅔ cup Honey Mustard Sauce (page 258)

Preheat the oven to 350 degrees F. Place the squash cut side down in a 2-inch-deep baking pan with ¼ inch of water. Bake them for 1 hour. Remove the squash from the oven and scrape out the insides with a fork—it will have a spaghettilike appearance. Put it in a serving bowl. Pour the sauce evenly over the squash and serve.

Yield: 4 servings (½ spaghetti squash per serving)

Each serving contains approximately: Calories 123 (7% from fat), Fat 1 g, Protein 1 g, Carbohydrate 29 g, Cholesterol 0 mg, Sodium 29 mg

Allowances: 2½ vegetables + 1 fruit

Spicy Thai Stir-Fry

> 1 teaspoon sesame oil
> 1 teaspoon extra-virgin olive oil
> 1 large red bell pepper, seeded and julienned
> 1 large onion, julienned
> 1 cup broccoli florets
> ½ cup mushrooms, stems removed and quartered
> ½ cup snow peas
> 1 teaspoon minced garlic
> 2 teaspoons minced ginger
> 4 ounces pineapple juice

1 jalapeño, seeded and diced
¼ cup chopped scallions

Heat a wok. Add the sesame and olive oils to the wok when it is hot. Then add the bell pepper and onion and sauté for 3 minutes. Add the broccoli and mushrooms and sauté for 3 minutes or more, constantly stirring the vegetables. Add all of the other ingredients except the scallions. Cook the vegetables for 1 minute longer. Remove from the heat. Top with the scallions and serve hot.

Yield: 4 servings (1 cup per serving)

Each serving contains approximately: Calories 74 (18% from fat), Protein 2.6 g, Fat 1.5 g, Carbohydrate 12 g, Cholesterol 0 mg, Sodium 10.6 mg

Allowances: ½ fat + 2 vegetables

Stuffed Cooked Tomatoes

1 teaspoon olive oil
4 large tomatoes
½ large onion, chopped
½ leek, chopped
¼ cup sliced mushrooms
1 teaspoon minced garlic
½ cup fresh, washed spinach
1 cup cooked rice (cooked in no-salt vegetable broth)
¼ cup no-salt tomato sauce (or marinara sauce)
1 teaspoon oregano
1 teaspoon basil
½ teaspoon thyme
1 teaspoon red pepper flates (optional)

Preheat the oven to 350 degrees F. Heat a large skillet over medium heat. Core the tomatoes and set aside. When the skillet is hot, add the olive oil, onions, and leek and sauté for a few minutes. Add the mushrooms and garlic and continue to sauté until the mushrooms are tender. Then add the spinach and continue to cook the vegetables for 3 to 5 more minutes. Remove from the heat. Mix the cooked rice in with the vegetables, along with the tomato sauce, herbs, and red pepper flakes, if using. Remove from the heat and stuff the cored tomatoes with the mixture. Place the stuffed tomatoes on a baking sheet and bake them in the oven for 20 to 25 minutes or until they are tender to the touch.

Yield: 4 servings (1 tomato per serving)

Each serving contains approximately: Calories 114 (16% from fat), Protein 3.5 g, Fat 2 g, Carbohydrate 22.2 g, Cholesterol 0 mg, Sodium 17 mg

Allowances: 1 starch + 1½ vegetables

Sweet Potato Burgers

    4 medium sweet potatoes
    1 small onion, diced
    ¼ cup diced green onions
    3 cloves garlic, minced
    2 tablespoons extra-virgin olive oil
    1 cup oats, finely ground in a food processor
    1 teaspoon ground cumin
    1 teaspoon lemon juice
    Parsley and cilantro (optional)

Preheat the oven to 400 degrees F. Bake the sweet potatoes for 45 minutes and let them cool. Reduce the oven temperature to 350 degrees F. Peel the sweet potatoes and set them aside. In a large pan, sauté the onions and garlic in olive oil over medium heat. In a large bowl, mix the sweet potatoes, onion, garlic, and all of the remaining ingredients except the parsley and cilantro. Form the mixture into 6 patties. In a hot skillet, pan-sear the burgers on both sides until they're brown, approximately 3 minutes on each side. Place them on a baking sheet and bake them for 10 minutes.

Chop the parsley and cilantro and garnish the top of each burger with both, if desired, creating a bed for the chili sauce and onions.

Chili Sauce

½ can (6 ounces) no-salt tomato paste
1 tablespoon chili powder
2 teaspoons garlic powder

Mix together all of the ingredients in a medium bowl.

Onion Topper

2 large onions
⅛ cup balsamic vinegar

Cut the onions into thin slices. Sauté the onions in the balsamic vinegar until they are translucent and most of the vinegar has cooked away, approximately 5 minutes.

Yield: 6 servings (1 patty with 1 cup sweet potato mixture + ⅙ of each topping, the chili sauce and onions, per serving)

Each serving contains approximately: Calories 183 (14% from fat), Protein 4.2 g, Fat 2.6 g, Carbohydrate 31.8 g, Cholesterol 0 mg, Sodium 37.8 mg

Allowances: 2 starches + ½ fat + ½ vegetable

Turkish Lentil-Tomato Soup

1 teaspoon extra-virgin olive oil
2 large onions, diced
2 large carrots, diced
2 teaspoons minced garlic
2 teaspoons ground cumin
2 teaspoons ground coriander
2 teaspoons ground fenugreek
½ teaspoon crushed red pepper flakes
2 large tomatoes, cored and chopped
1 cup red lentils (soaked overnight)

5 cups no-salt vegetable stock
¼ cup fresh dill

Heat a medium sauté pan over medium-high heat, then add the olive oil. Add the onions and carrots and sauté them until they're tender. Add the garlic and the remaining herbs. Add the tomatoes and simmer everything for 10 minutes. Transfer the ingredients to a soup pot. Add the lentils and vegetable stock. Cover the pot and cook on low heat until the lentils are soft, approximately 30 minutes. Remove the pot from the heat and place the mixture into a blender or a food processor. Puree the ingredients until they're smooth. Stir in half of the dill. Garnish the soup with the remaining dill, if desired. Serve hot.

Yield: 6 servings (1 cup per serving)

Each serving contains approximately: Calories 197 (14% from fat), Protein 11 g, Fat 3.1 g, Carbohydrate 23.3 g, Cholesterol 0 mg, Sodium 37.1 mg

Allowances: ¼ fat + 2 starches + 1 vegetable

White Beans and Greens

1 tablespoon extra-virgin olive oil
6–8 cloves of garlic, chopped
2 pounds seasonal greens (escarole, mustard greens, turnip greens, broccoli rabe, dandelion greens, kale, chard, and beet greens all work well), chopped
1 can no-salt white beans of choice; great northern or cannellini are best (if using dry beans, approximately 1½ cups of cooked beans is equivalent to 1 can)
2 tablespoons no-salt vegetable stock or water
Juice of 1 lemon

Heat a large sauté pan over medium-high heat, then add the olive oil. Add the garlic and sauté until it's tender. Add the chopped greens to the sauté pan, moving the greens constantly with tongs. Allow the garlic to disperse through the greens. Add the beans and vegetable stock. Let the mixture simmer until the greens are cooked through. Squeeze the lemon juice over the beans and greens mixture and serve over rice or pasta.

Yield: 6 servings (1 cup per serving)

Each serving contains approximately: Calories 120 (23% from fat), Protein 8 g, Fat 3 g, Carbohydrate 19 g, Cholesterol 0 mg, Sodium 32 mg

Allowances: ¾ starch + 1½ vegetables + ½ fat

Appendix A
Grocery and Staples Lists

The following foods can be obtained at your local farmer's market, food co-op, community support agriculture (CSA) organization, and grocery stores; remember, local organic is best. A detailed grocery list for each of the seasonal menu plans can be found at www.ricediet.com. (NAS = no added salt.)

Grocery List
- Bananas
- Pears, organic
- Apples, organic
- Dried fruit: prunes, cherries, raisins, mangos
- Grapefruit
- Tangerines
- Cauliflower
- Peppers, organic
- Baby carrots, organic
- Celery, organic
- Salmon (wild-caught, frozen) or any fresh, local fish
- Favorite fresh herbs: parsley, sage, rosemary, thyme, cilantro, basil, oregano
- Broccoli sprouts or clover sprouts
- Yogurt, organic, nonfat, plain
- Soy milk, organic, plain
- Granola
- Tofu and tempeh, NAS
- Local, organically grown lean meats (if risk factors suggest it is appropriate for you to eat meat)

- Kashi Cinnamon Harvest (shredded wheat)
- Walnuts, almonds, pumpkin and sesame seeds*

Pantry Staples
- Oat groats or oatmeal, grits
- Rice (brown), barley, quinoa, faro, polenta, kasha (buckwheat groats)
- Dried Beans (black, navy, pinto, cannellini)
- Bean Cuisine Soup mixes (can be found at www.ricediet.com)
- Dried pasta (penne, angel hair; my favorites are fregola and strozzapreti)
- Panko bread crumbs
- Extra-virgin olive oil
- Balsamic vinegar
- Honey (local)
- Canned beans: black, garbanzo, organic, NAS
- Tomatoes, canned, organic, NAS
- Tomato sauce and tomato paste, NAS
- Muir Glen Fire Roasted Diced Tomatoes
- Salsa, NAS (e.g., Enrico's)
- Dessert Pepper Tuscan White Bean Dip
- Sardines and tuna, NAS
- Garlic and onions
- Favorite dried spices and herbs
- Vegetable bouillon, NAS
- Lemons and limes
- Green tea and other favorite teas
- Nutritional yeast

Freezer Staples
- NAS bread (like Ezekiel Bread or Toufayan pita bread; contact 800-EAT-PITA)
- Grapes and blueberries
- Vegetables, NAS (e.g., Bird's Eye artichoke hearts)

---

* Items that may inspire excessive consumption can be purchased in small amounts (e.g., nuts and cheese). Nuts can be purchased in bulk, a quarter cup at a time; the cheese counter employee can slice small portions of cheese and rewrap it.

Farmer's Market

- Fresh vegetables: include a variety of colorful dark orange, red and green vegetables, such as baby greens, arugula, tomatoes, and fresh herbs
- Eggs, free-range, organic

Appendix B
Assessing the True Cost of
Your Food

You are on a mission to buy the freshest, healthiest foods, primarily organic and locally grown, for at least four days of menu planning. Since the largest selection of organic and locally grown foods would be available at your farmer's market, food co-op, or community-supported agriculture farm, you may want to start your shopping excursion at one of these sources. But if a chain grocery store is your only choice, remember that you can politely ask the produce manager the geographical source of the product you desire.

Questions to ask the farmer purveyor:

> Is he or she certified organic? Why or why not? Does he or she follow organic farming practices but choose not to pay the costly fees associated with certification?
> How far (in miles) did the food travel today?
> If the food in question is animal in origin, such as eggs, dairy, or meat, what was the animal fed? Ask whether genetically modified corn was used in the feed.

Although produce managers may not know the specifics about the food they sell, they certainly would benefit by learning more about their products. It is not too much to ask them to check the case container to find out where a product was grown. Although initially this may feel challenging, it is an education for both you and the produce manager and will be very enlightening.

Resources

Music

This book is complemented by the musical CD, *Healing at the Roots and Sounds of Renewal*, a collaborative work performed and produced by Little Windows. The CD can be purchased at www.ricediet.com or www.littlewindows.net.

If you have not seen the award-winning documentary *Playing for Change: Peace through Music* with many musicians performing the song "Stand by Me," please visit www.flixxy.com/peace-through-music.htm.

You may also want to check out the following:

Wintley Phipps's performance of "Amazing Grace" at www.youtube .com/watch?v=HfGytXRpfho

Joshua Bell's classical violin performance in a Washington, D.C., subway at: www.washingtonpost.com/wp-dyn/content/article/2007/04/04/ AR2007040401721.html

More than two hundred dancers performing their version of "Do Re Mi" in the Central Station of Antwerp, Belgium, another fun multisensory experience in connecting creatively, at www.youtube .com/watch?v=7EYAUazLI9k

Practitioners

Todd Brazee, breath therapist, toddbrazee@hotmail.com. Todd works in private practice in Santa Monica and Malibu, California, and is also involved in university research projects relating to the reduction of severity of trauma and addiction symptomology. His work also includes nationwide lectures, experiential workshops, and private session tours. Todd travels throughout the country to work with individuals and families suffering from emotional trauma.

Karen Winstead, practitioner of axiatonal attunement, is associated with the Institute for Research and Development of Alternative Healing. To learn more about her, visit www.innersoulutions.org). She can also be reached at (828) 773–7556.

Carolyn Craft has years of experience as a minister, counselor, broadcaster, speaker, corporate executive, and spiritual leader and brings many skills to her work at the Rice Diet Program. From her years of interviewing nationally known leaders in the holistic field, from Deepak Chopra to Caroline Myss, to her facilitation of Nonviolent Communication, Hakomi Therapy, Mindfulness Practice, and HeartMath Techniques, she counsels with great wisdom. Carolyn has a private spiritual counseling practice in Durham, North Carolina, and can be reached at www.carolyncraft.com and (919) 612–8899.

Food

To procure locally grown, organic foods and stay informed, visit these Web sites:

www.organ-center.org

www.seedsofdeception.com

www.ewg.org

www.foodincmovie.com

www.ams.usda.gov/
   farmersmarkets

www.localharvest.org

www.cornucopia.org

www.organicconsumers.org

www.responsibletechnology.org

www.endhunger.org

DVDs

These DVDs provide a true education on the condition of our food supply:

Food, Inc.

The Future of Food

Unnatural Selection

Our Daily Bread

The Greening of Cuba

Fresh

These two DVDs will educate you on the power of intention:

What the Bleep Do We Know!?

The Secret

Books and CDs

Gary Craig's *The EFT Manual*, 6th ed., is available for free at www.emofree.com.

Francis and Judith MacNutt, *School of Healing Prayer: Level I* (12-CD set). You may order it from Christian Healing Ministries, Inc., P.O. Box 9520, Jacksonville, FL 32208; (904) 765–3332; www.christianhealingmin.org.

Jon Kabat-Zinn, *Mindfulness Meditation* practice CDs and tapes, series 1, 2, and 3. Your may order them from www.mindfulnesstapes.com or ricediet.com, or by mail from Stress Reduction Tapes, P.O. Box 547, Lexington, MA 02420.

Thich Nhat Hahn, *Plum Village Meditations: With Thich Nhat Hahn and Sister Jina Van Hengel*. Louisville, CO: Sounds True, 1997.

Bernie Siegel, *Faith, Hope and Healing: Inspiring Lessons Learned from People Living with Cancer; Love, Medicine and Miracles: Lessons Learned about Self-Healing from a Surgeon's Experience with Exceptional Patients;* and 365 *Prescriptions for the Soul: Daily Messages of Inspiration, Hope, and Love*.

Organic and Biodynamic Seeds

Seeds of Change (seedsofchange.com) has 100 percent certified organic seed types and over twelve hundred varieties, with many heirloom, native, and hard to find seeds.

Seed Alliance (seedalliance.org) can assist you in finding many different organic seed suppliers.

Turtle Tree Seed (turtletreeseed.com) is a biodynamic seed initiative that sells flower, vegetable, and herb seeds.

Web Sites

These sites will lead you to products that will help you strengthen your body, stay flexible, and assist with relieving muscle spasms and pain.

Premium Eva Foam Roller: Help with releasing lower back spasms. For more information, visit www.power-systems.com/p-2972-premium-eva-foam-roller.aspx.

Yamuna Body Rolling: A health and fitness therapy that creates positive, long-lasting changes in your body using specially designed balls and other aids. For more information, call 800-877-8429 or visit www.yamunabodyrolling.com.

References

Books

With respect for the trees and the energy required to print the full list of references, some primary ones will be listed below and the entirety will be available at www.ricediet.com.

Barks, Coleman, trans. *The Essential Rumi*. New York: HarperOne, 2004.

Begley, Sharon. *Train Your Mind: Change Your Brain*. New York: Ballantine Books, 2007.

Bittman, Mark. *Food Matters: A Guide to Conscious Eating*. New York: Simon and Schuster, 2009.

Buettner, Dan. *The Blue Zones: Lessons for Living Longer from the People Who've Lived the Longest*. New York: Random House, 2009.

Capacchione, Lucia. *The Power of Your Other Hand: A Course in Channeling the Inner Wisdom of the Right Brain*. North Hollywood, CA: Newcastle Publishing, 1988.

Dossey, Larry. *Healing Words*. New York: HarperCollins, 1993.

Fredrickson, Barbara L. *Positivity: Groundbreaking Research Reveals How to Embrace the Hidden Strength of Positive Emotions, Overcome Negativity, and Thrive*. New York: Crown Publishers, 2009.

Hay, Louise. *You Can Heal Your Life*. Carlsbad, CA: Hay House, 1984.

Hill, Napoleon. *Think and Grow Rich*. Revised and expanded by Arthur R. Pell. New York: Penguin, 2005.

Jampolsky, G. G. *Love Is Letting Go of Fear*. New York: Ten Speed Press, 2004.

Keating, Thomas. *Open Mind Open Heart: The Contemplative Dimension of the Gospel*. New York: Continuum, 1986.

Kelsey, Morton T. *Dreams: A Way to Listen to God.* New York: Paulist Press, 1978.

——. *Psychology, Medicine and Christian Healing.* San Francisco: Harper & Row, 1988.

Kingsolver, Barbara, Camille Kingsolver, and Steven L. Hopp. *Animal, Vegetable, Miracle: A Year of Food Life.* New York: HarperCollins, 2007.

Koenig, H. *The Healing Power of Faith: Science Explores Medicine's Last Great Frontier.* New York: Simon and Schuster, 1999.

Lee, Victoria. *The Rumi Secret: Spiritual Lessons of History's Most Revered Poet.* Denver, CO: Outskirts Press, 2007.

Levitin, Daniel J. *This Is Your Brain on Music: The Science of a Human Obsession.* New York: Plume, 2007.

MacNutt, Francis. *Healing.* Notre Dame, IN: Ave Maria Press, 1985.

Pert, Candace B. *Molecules of Emotion: The Science behind Mind-Body Medicine.* New York: Simon and Schuster, 1997.

Smith, J. *Genetic Roulette: The Documented Health Risks of Genetically Engineered Foods.* Fairfield, IA: Yes! Books, 2007.

Steiner, Rudolf. *What Is Biodynamics? A Way to Heal and Revitalize the Earth.* Great Barrington, MA: SteinerBooks, 2005.

Journal and Web Site Articles

Beck, R. J., T. C. Cesario, A. Yousefi, and H. Enamoto. "Choral Singing, Performance Perception, and Immune System Changes in Salivary Immunoglobulin A and Cortisol." *Music Perception,* 18, no. 1 (2001), 87–106.

Benbrook, C., and A. Greene. "The Link Between Organic and Health: New Research Makes the Case for Organic Even Stronger." *Organic Processing Magazine,* January–February 2008.

Boden, W. E., et al. "Impact of Optimal Medical Therapy with or without Percutaneous Coronary Intervention on Long-Term Cardiovascular End Points in Patients with Stable Coronary Artery Disease (from the COURAGE Trial)." *American Journal of Cardiology* 104, no. 1 (2009): 1–4.

CDC Morbidity and Mortality Weekly Report. "Application of Lower Sodium Intake Recommendations to Adults—United States, 1999–2006." March 27, 2009, www.cdc.gov/mmwr/preview/mmwrhtml/mm5811a2.htm.

Coylewright, M., R. S. Blumenthal, and W. Post. "Placing COURAGE in Context: Review of the Recent Literature on Managing Stable Coronary Artery Disease." *Mayo Clinic Proceedings* 83, no. 7 (2008): 799–805.

Department of Veterinary Medicine, FDA, correspondence, June 16, 1993, as quoted in Fred A. Hines, memo to Dr. Linda Kahl. "Flavr Savr Tomato: Pathology Branch's Evaluation of Rats with Stomach Lesions from Three Four-Week Oral (Gavage) Toxicity Studies and an Expert Panel's Report." Alliance for Bio-Integrity, June 16, 1993, www.biointegrity.org/FDAdocs/17/view1.html.

Ewen, Stanley W. B., and Arpad Pusztai. "Effect of Diets Containing Genetically Modified Potatoes Expressing Galanthus Nivalis Lectin on Rat Small Intestine." *Lancet* (October 16, 1999): 1353–1354.

Fares, Nagui H., and Adel K. El-Sayed. "Fine Structural Changes in the Ileum of Mice Fed on Endotoxin-Treated Potatoes and Transgenic Potatoes." *Natural Toxins* 6, no. 6 (1998): 219–233.

Fonseca-Alaniz, M. H., Luciana D. Brito, Christina N. Borges-Silva, et al. "High Dietary Sodium Intake Increases White Adipose Tissue Mass and Plasma Leptin in Rats." *Obesity* 15, no. 9 (September 2007): 2200–2208.

GM Watch (EU). "New Study Links Genetically Engineered Corn to Infertility." Organic Consumers Web site, November 12, 2008, www.organicconsumers.org/articles/article_15588.cfm.

Johnson, Carl B., to Linda Kahl and others. "Flavr Savr™ Tomato: Significance of Pending DHEE Question." Alliance for Bio-Integrity, December 7, 1993, www.biointegrity.org.

Jacobson, Michael F. "Tackling Salt." *Nutrition Action Healthletter,* January–February 2008.

Monsanto vs. U.S. Farmers. A Report by the Center for Food Safety, 2005. http://truefoodnow.files.wordpress.com/2009/12/cfsmonsantovsfarmerreport1-13-05.pdf.

Pusztai, Arpad. "Genetically Modified Foods: Are They a Risk to Human/Animal Health?" *Action Bioscience*, June 2001, www.actionbioscience.org/biotech/pusztai.html.

———. "Facts behind the GM Pea Controversy: Epigenetics, Transgenic Plants and Risk Assessment." Proceedings of the Conference, December 1, 2005. Frankfurt: Literaturhaus, 2005.

Reuters. "GMO Corn Causes Liver, Kidney Problems in Rats: Study" (regarding the study published in the peer-reviewed journal *Archives of Environmental Contamination and Technology*). March 13, 2007, www.reuters.com/article/environmentNews/idUSL134684002 0070314.

Rosati, R. A., et al. "Does Coronary Surgery Prolong Life in Comparison with Medical Management?" *Postgraduate Medical Journal* 52 (2007): 749–756.

Scheuplein, Robert J. Memo to the FDA Biotechnology Coordinator and others. "Response to Calgene Amended Petition." Alliance for Bio-Integrity, October 27, 1993, www.biointegrity.org.

Index

Page numbers in *italics* refer to illustrations and photos.